Camila Araújo Bernardino Garcia

Neuroprotective effects of Edaravone in experimental hydrocephalus

Camila Araújo Bernardino Garcia

Neuroprotective effects of Edaravone in experimental hydrocephalus

In young Wistar rats induced with hydrocephalus via kaolin

ScienciaScripts

Imprint
Any brand names and product names mentioned in this book are subject to trademark, brand or patent protection and are trademarks or registered trademarks of their respective holders. The use of brand names, product names, common names, trade names, product descriptions etc. even without a particular marking in this work is in no way to be construed to mean that such names may be regarded as unrestricted in respect of trademark and brand protection legislation and could thus be used by anyone.

Cover image: www.ingimage.com

This book is a translation from the original published under ISBN 978-3-330-76288-6.

Publisher:
Sciencia Scripts
is a trademark of
Dodo Books Indian Ocean Ltd. and OmniScriptum S.R.L publishing group

120 High Road, East Finchley, London, N2 9ED, United Kingdom
Str. Armeneasca 28/1, office 1, Chisinau MD-2012, Republic of Moldova, Europe
Managing Directors: Ieva Konstantinova, Victoria Ursu
info@omniscriptum.com

Printed at: see last page
ISBN: 978-620-8-38997-0

DEDICATORY

To my dear mum Márcia Cassis for her love and tireless encouragement.

ACKNOWLEDGEMENTS

Luiza da Silva Lopes

He taught and instructed me without reservation throughout this stage, always willing to recommend readings and carry out the practical part. I would like to thank her for the generous way in which she guided me through this work and for her support during my professional and personal development.

Hélio Rubens Machado

For his example of character and professionalism, his sensitivity in saying the right words at the right times helped me to steer my research and awaken my scientific outlook. I am immensely grateful to you for trusting me and always motivating my intellectual development.

To my friends and lab mates

To all my friends in the lab, for the days of work shared with joy and good humour. Many thanks to everyone for their dedication and understanding during stressful times.

USP guest house - Ribeirão Preto campus

To the staff who welcomed me with so much affection and attention every school day!

Staff of the Department of Surgery and Anatomy

For their support, care and willingness to help whenever necessary. I thank you for all your affection.

FAEPA - Foundation for the Support of Teaching, Research and Assistance at the Hospital das Clínicas, Ribeirão Preto Medical School, University of São Paulo

Financial support for the congresses and events I attended.

FAPESP - São Paulo Research Foundation

For the grant and financial support to carry out this research.

To everyone I share the joy of having done this work.

SPECIAL THANKS

To my family

To my parents Mauro Bemardino and Márcia Cassis, an example of success and unconditional love. Thank you so much for your support in difficult times, for your encouragement and, above all, for motivating me to be an honest and hard-working person. To my sister Marcela Araújo, confidant and companion, who was always by my side, suffering with me the nerves of the pre-presentations and selections to enrol in the postgraduate programme. To my husband Marlon Garcia, the great love of my life, who with great affection and complicity has always encouraged me, believed in my professional growth and understood my absence from home because I live in another city, dedicating myself to my studies, with tireless companionship! I love you all!

Summary

Introduction: Hydrocephalus is a syndrome characterised by the accumulation of cerebrospinal fluid inside the ventricular cavities. Considering its multifactorial pathophysiology, one of the factors involved is oxidative stress triggered by lipid peroxidation and the formation of free radicals. Edaravone is a new antioxidant drug with neuroprotective effects that has not yet been tested in patients with hydrocephalus. **Aim: To** evaluate the neuroprotective response of Edaravone in experimental hydrocephalus in young rats. **Methodology:** Hydrocephalus was induced in young rats by injecting a portion of kaolin into the cisterna magna. The animals were divided into three groups: control (C) (n=10); untreated hydrocephalus (HNT) (n=20); hydrocephalus treated with 20mg/kg Edaravone (HTE) (n=20). The drug-treated group received an intraperitoneal injection of Edaravone every day from the first day after induction. The animals were weighed daily, assessed by behavioural tests and magnetic resonance imaging, histopathological analysis, immunohistochemistry and biochemistry. All the animals were sacrificed, 14 days after the induction of hydrocephalus. **Results:** From the third to the eighth day after hydrocephalus induction, the animals gained less weight than the controls. However, from the ninth day after induction, weight gain was similar in the three experimental groups. In the open field test and the water maze, the performance of the animals in the HTE group was better when compared to the animals in the HNT group. In immunohistochemistry for GFAP, the animals in the HNT group showed intensely labelled astrocytes with thick extensions, while the animals in the HTE group had more delicate astrocytes with thin extensions. In the caspase-3 analysis, the animals treated with Edaravone showed a lower number of cells undergoing apoptosis. **Conclusions:** The use of Edaravone showed a tendency to reduce cells undergoing apoptosis, improved behavioural response, and slightly reduced astrocyte activity as evidenced by GFAP immunolabelling in the corpus callosum of young rats with hydrocephalus.

Keywords: experimental hydrocephalus, neuroprotection, Edaravone.

Summary

CHAPTER 1

INTRODUCTION

Hydrocephalus is a disease with a complex pathophysiology, which not only affects the dynamics of cerebrospinal fluid (CSF), but also other structures of the central nervous system. The imbalance between CSF production and absorption results in an increase in ventricular volume and leads to distortions in the brain parenchyma, compressing the hemispheres against the inner surface of the skull (DEL BIGIO; BRUNI; FEWER, 1985).

Various classifications attempt to define hydrocephalus using different criteria, and no classification is complete and satisfactory. As for the pathological processes, they can be of acute or chronic development. In addition, hydrocephalus can also be classified according to the point at which the cerebrospinal fluid circulation is blocked, into non-communicating, when the blockage is within the ventricular system, and communicating, when the blockage is outside the ventricular system, affecting the cisterns at the base of the brain, or other points in the subarachnoid space, or even the arachnoid villi. Hydrocephalus can be caused by obstruction of the cerebrospinal fluid pathways or by overproduction of cerebrospinal fluid. These two basic causes can be triggered by neoplasms, congenital malformations or inflammatory processes (MILHORAT, 1979).

Normal cerebrospinal fluid production in an adult male is around 500 ml per day. As the cerebrospinal fluid space holds between 130 and 140 ml, there is a total exchange of cerebrospinal fluid 3 or 4 times a day (MCLONE, 1994). In hydrocephalus, with altered cerebrospinal fluid dynamics and the accumulation of cerebrospinal fluid in the dilated ventricular system, there is stagnation and impaired elimination of metabolites (CASTRO-GAGO *et al.,* 1989). With the accumulation of cerebrospinal fluid in the ventricular cavities, intracranial pressure rises, especially in the acute stages of obstructive hydrocephalus. However, the increase in intracranial pressure is not the only factor involved in the genesis of ventricular dilatation. This can be seen in normal pressure hydrocephalus, in which intracranial pressure, apparently compensated, returns to normal values during the development of the process, without preventing ventricular dilation from progressing. It is probably the pressure gradient between the ventricles and the brain parenchyma that actually leads to dilation (SATO; OI; YAMADA, 1999).

Due to its proximity to the ventricular cavity, the first structure to be affected is the ependyma, which suffers compression and stretching, and these alterations can lead to the destruction of this epithelium, at isolated points or even its total rupture. The changes to the choroid plexus are milder than those to the ependyma, with distortion of the villi, flattening and vacuolisation of the cells, formation of intracellular inclusions and widening of the intercellular spaces (KIEFER *et al.*, 1998). The white matter also suffers the consequences of ventricular dilation, with regional differences, depending on the age of onset of hydrocephalus, which in more pronounced degrees of ventricular dilation shows a loss of myelin content. Myelin damage can also be the result of oedema, as cerebrospinal fluid contains proteolytic enzymes (MABE; SUZUKI; NAGAI, 1990).

Later, astrogliosis occurs, replacing the damaged axons and myelin (DEL BIGIO; MCALLISTER II, 1999). In more extreme degrees of ventricular dilation, the corpus callosum can be completely destroyed (SHOESMITH; BUIST; DEL BIGIO, 2000). The distortion of the brain leads to stretching and distortion of the cerebral vessels, as well as a reduction in the density of the capillaries, resulting in a drop in cerebral blood flow (PORTNOY; BRANCH; CASTRO, 1994).

Hydrocephalus also affects neurons and compromises synapses. The neuronal body may show chromatolysis and vacuolisation and the dendrites may be shortened and reduced in number, with fewer dendritic spicules. Cortical compression causes packing of the neurons, with a reduction in size and rounding or flattening of the pyramidal neurons (EDWARDS *et al.*, 1984, KHAN; ENNO; DEL BIGIO, 2006). Other structures, such as the hippocampus, basal nuclei, cerebellum and thalamus, show only slight alterations, with their neurons more preserved.

1.1. Epidemiology

Hydrocephalus is an extremely important problem for clinical and surgical neurology. It is one of the most common diseases affecting the central nervous system (CNS) during the neonatal period and infancy.

Worldwide incidences of congenital hydrocephalus range from 0.3 to 1.0/1,000 births. The non-communicating form, however, reaches rates of 1.0 to 3.0/1,000 (JULIAN-REYNIER *et al.*, 1994). Another source, following studies carried out in four European regions, published a prevalence of 4.65/10,000 live births (GARNE *et al.*, 2010).

A survey carried out between 1997 and 2000 showed that of the total volume of surgeries at the Neurosurgery Service of the Hospital das Clínicas of the Ribeirão Preto-USP Medical School, 29 per cent were related to CSF shunt implants and revisions, and 35 per cent of the patients operated on were under two years old. However, surgical procedures can account for up to 60% of the turnover of an exclusively paediatric neurosurgery service (JUCÁ *et al.*, 2002).

Epidemiological information from the National Health Service of the United States of America (USA) recorded more than 125,000 cerebrospinal fluid shunts performed in 1995. Of all these procedures, 33,000 resulted in the placement of a valve to treat hydrocephalus. The country spends an estimated 100 million dollars a year on tests alone to diagnose and direct the appropriate therapeutic approach, while the cost involved in treating hydrocephalus varies according to the shunt system chosen, the use of medication, especially antibiotics, as well as surgeries and the length of hospitalisation for these procedures (BONDURANT; JIMENEZ, 1995).

1.2. Experimental hydrocephalus

For research purposes, it was necessary to develop experimental methods with the aim of understanding the pathophysiology of hydrocephalus and developing possible treatment techniques. Kaolin is a chemically inert substance, composed of treated aluminium silicate, which causes an inflammatory process in the meninges, obstructing the exit of the fourth ventricle, without directly damaging the brain parenchyma and without causing inflammation of the subarachnoid space (DEFEO *et al.,* 1979, EDWARDS *et al.*, 1984, HOCHWALD, 1985).

Dixon and Heller (1932) published the first study using kaolin to produce experimental hydrocephalus. Injection of kaolin into the cisterna magna has been shown to induce non-communicating hydrocephalus which, in the acute stage, is characterised by increased intracranial pressure and progressive ventriculomegaly. In the chronic stage, intracranial pressure normalises and ventricular dilation stabilises (BRAUN *etal.,* 1998).

The production of hydrocephalus by intracistemal injection of kaolin has been successfully carried out in experimental animals (dogs, cats, rats and mice). One study with mice successfully induced hydrocephalus by percutaneous injection of kaolin into the cisterna magna, both in young adults and in seven-day-old animals. The authors studied the effects of the disease by assessing behavioural and histological changes in these animals (LOPES; SLOBODIAN; DEL BIGIO, 2009).

Different methods of producing experimental hydrocephalus have disadvantages in relation to kaolin, as they require extensive surgical procedures and can cause undesirable anatomical changes. The results often fail, either because they cause fulminant hydrocephalus or because the rate of hydrocephalus production is very low. In addition, these methods do not represent the natural pathological process in most cases of hydrocephalus, unlike kaolin, which produces an inflammatory reaction similar to that seen in humans with hydrocephalus after infection or subarachnoid haemorrhage (DEFEO *etal.,* 1979, EDWARDS *et al.,* 1984).

Recently, strains of animals genetically susceptible to hydrocephalus have been used (LEE *et al.,* 2002, VOGEL *et al.,* 2012). These animals present hydrocephalus during intrauterine development, preventing the choice of the beginning of ventricular dilation, as well as not guaranteeing that the alterations found are purely a consequence of hydrocephalus and not the genetic malformation itself, reducing the possibility of study depending on the research objective.

Due to the factors present in the different methods mentioned above, we opted to use kaolin because it is more efficient, has a lower financial cost, does not require surgical procedures and does not lead to alterations other than those resulting from hydrocephalus.

1.3. Oxidative stress

The human body is constantly affected by reactive oxygen species (ROS) and reactive nitrogen species (RNS), which are generated by inflammatory processes, biological dysfunction or food. The main ROS fall into two groups: radical (hydroxyl, superoxide, peroxyl and alkoxyl) and non-radical (oxygen, hydrogen peroxide and hypochlorous acid). ERNS include nitric oxide, nitrous oxide, nitrous acid, nitrites, nitrates and peroxynitrites. While some of them can be highly reactive in the body, attacking lipids, proteins and DNA, others are only reactive with lipids. There are also some that are not very reactive, but can nevertheless generate harmful species. The radical is the most harmful to the organism, because due to its half-life it can hardly be sequestered *in vivo* (HALLIWELL, 2007).

There is great interest in studying the effect of oxidative stress due to discoveries about the action of antioxidants. Oxidation is a fundamental part of aerobic life and our metabolism, so free radicals are produced naturally or by some biological dysfunction.

These free radicals, whose unpaired electrons are centred on oxygen or nitrogen atoms, which are EROS in the body, are involved in energy production, phagocytosis, cell growth regulation, intercellular signalling and the synthesis of important biological substances. However, their excess has harmful effects, such as lipid peroxidation and damage to tissue and membrane proteins, which are related to various pathologies, such as arthritis, haemorrhagic shock, heart disease, cataracts, cognitive dysfunction, cancer and AIDS, and may be the cause or aggravating factor of the general condition (HUSAIN *et al., 1987).*

Oxidative stress is present in hydrocephalus due to the aggression caused to the brain parenchyma by compression and stretching forces. This action leads to tissue damage, with the production of free radicals, mainly through lipid peroxidation, which has a toxic effect on the walls of cerebral arterial vessels (CANER *et al.,* 1993, FERSTEN *et al.,* 2004).

Excess free radicals in the body are combated by antioxidants produced by the body or absorbed from the diet. Antioxidants are defined as any substance which, present in lower concentrations than the oxidisable substrate, is capable of effectively delaying or inhibiting oxidation. These substances can act directly, neutralising the action of free radicals and non-radical species, or indirectly, participating in enzyme systems with this capacity (SIES, 1997).

The antioxidant defence system has the function of inhibiting and/or reducing the damage caused by the deleterious action of free radicals or reactive non-radical species. These actions can be achieved through different mechanisms of action, preventing the formation of free radicals or non-radical species (prevention systems), preventing their action (scavenging systems) or favouring the repair and reconstitution of damaged biological structures (repair systems) (DEVARAJ *et al.,* 2007).

The non-enzymatic mechanism is made up of a wide variety of antioxidant substances, which can be endogenous or dietary in origin. Glutathione is an essential tripeptide made up of three amino acids: glycine, glutamic acid and cysteine. The synthesis of this tripeptide (y-glutamylcysteinylglycine) occurs from a reaction catalysed by the enzyme y-glutamylcysteine synthetase (y-GCS), which uses glutamate and cysteine to give rise to y-glutamylcysteine, which together with glycine, through a reaction catalysed by glutathione synthetase, will form glutathione (DRINGEN; GUTTERER; HIRRLINGER, 2000). With endogenous antioxidant action, found in all animal cells, it reacts with free radicals and can protect tissues from damage caused by singlet oxygen and hydroxide and superoxide radicals. In trauma, there is a reduction in the level of glutathione, secondary to oxidative stress (HALLIWELL; WHITEMAN, 2004).

There are currently many doubts about the molecular mechanisms responsible for the pathophysiology of hydrocephalus. Several studies have attempted to establish a relationship between hydrocephalus and oxidative stress. In the study carried out by Mori et al. (1993) on congenital hydrocephalus in the brains of adult WIC-HYD rats, immunohistochemical analysis revealed a reduction in the enzyme superoxide dismutase (SOD) in the ependyma, choroid plexus and hippocampus. In kaolin-induced hydrocephalus in rats, lipid peroxide levels can increase after the induction of hydrocephalus (CANER *et al.,* 1993). Six-week-old hydrocephalic rats had a significant increase in EROS levels, after treatment with an antioxidant drug, the animals increased their levels of FOXO3a +/- FANCD2 +/-, indicating protection against cell death through the use of the antioxidant and a significant reduction in the death of the hydrocephalic pups (LI, X. *et al.,* 2014).

1.4. Neuroprotection and Edaravone

Neuroprotection can be defined as an intervention, not necessarily pharmacological, but directly linked to the intracellular mechanisms of the ischaemic cascade, aimed at rescuing the still viable area of hypoperfusion surrounding the infarct (area of necrosis). It encompasses measures that improve the blood supply to the tissue and measures that increase the viability of the cell in the face of reduced circulation (ZAGER; AMES, 1988, ATES *et al.*, 2007).

The drug MCI-186 (3-methyl-l-phenyl-2-pyrazolin-5-one) also called Edaravone is a synthetic free radical scavenger that was approved in Japan in April 2001 for the treatment of acute cerebral infarction. It has an inhibitory effect on lipid peroxidation by scavenging free radicals and has been used to reduce neuronal damage after ischaemic stroke (ISHIBASHI; YOSHITAKE; ADACHI, 2013, KIKUCHI *et al.*, 2013, DOHARE *et al.*, 2014).

The main focus of research into Edaravone is its potential as a free radical scavenger, as it has a low molecular weight and can easily cross the blood-brain barrier (WATANABE; TAHARA; TODO, 2008). Under physiological conditions, with a neutral pH, Edaravone is present in an anionic form, i.e. its metabolisation in the body occurs through a process of electron transfer. These are released from Edaravone and can eliminate radical species containing a free electron, such as a peroxide-lipid radical, which is formed after the extraction of a free radical proton from an unsaturated fatty acid (HIGASHI *et al.*, 2006).

Edaravone's therapeutic benefit may go beyond its antioxidant activity. Its multi-target pharmacology means that it has the ability to regulate other signalling pathways. For example, recent research has suggested that Edaravone can suppress neuronal death (YOSHIDA *et al.*, 2006), neutralise neurotoxicity in microglia (BANNO *et al.*, 2005) and reduce long-term inflammation (ZHANG *et al.*, 2005).

Edaravone has been shown to prevent the development of oedema following a stroke by inhibiting astrogliosis and the expression of vascular endothelial growth factor (ISHIKAWA *et al.*, 2007).

A study using an ischaemia and reperfusion model in rodents provided additional evidence that Edaravone reduced the damage caused by ischaemia (WU *et* a/.,2000).

Other studies have also shown that Edaravone can inhibit lipoxygenase, an enzyme responsible for lipid oxidation (HIGASHI *et al.*, 2006) but can also directly suppress the oxidation of low density lipoproteins (YOSHIDA *etal.*, 2006).

Using a population of stroke patients, researchers studied the effects of Edaravone on functional outcome. An important difference to note in this study is the length of hospital stay and improvement in motor paralysis. Statistical analysis shows that there was a greater reduction in the average length of hospitalisation and motor rehabilitation in the group treated with Edaravone when compared to the untreated group (OHTA *et al.,* 2009).

A study on internal carotid artery occlusion in patients also showed the efficacy of Edaravone. Mortality in the acute post-occlusion phase decreased in the treated group, with 20% mortality compared to 45% mortality in the untreated group. Considering the devastating nature of stroke, these results are significant (TOYODA *etal.,* 2004).

In addition to cerebral ischaemia, its neuroprotective effect has been proven in other neurological diseases, such as neonatal encephalopathy (NAKAMURA *et al.*, 2008) acute intracerebral haemorrhage (NOOR *et al.*, 2005), (YAGI *et al.,* 2009), subarachnoid haemorrhage (MUNAKATA *et al.,* 2009), amyotrophic lateral sclerosis (ITO *et al.*, 2008), traumatic brain injury (ITOH *et al*., 2009), spinal cord injury (WANG *et al.*, 2013), epilepsy (KAMIDA *et al.,* 2009). In an experimental model of cerebral thrombosis and treatment with Edaravone, it was associated with functional recovery of hemiparesis, and reduction of the infarct area (INOUE *etal.*, 2014).

CHAPTER 2

BACKGROUND

As not all patients can undergo surgical treatment with cerebrospinal fluid *shunts* immediately after diagnosis, either because they have unfavourable clinical conditions or because they still have initial ventricular dilatation, neuroprotective drugs are being tested in an attempt to reduce tissue damage until definitive treatment, or even to reinforce complete recovery after the installation of a *shunt.*

CHAPTER 3

OBJECTIVES

To evaluate the neuroprotective response of Edaravone in experimental hydrocephalus,

through:

- Behavioural tests: open field (to assess sensorimotor development) and Morris water maze (to assess memory and learning).
- Magnetic resonance imaging of the brain: to determine the degree of ventriculomegaly (ventricular ratio) and the degree of cerebral myelination (magnetisation transfer).
- Histology: haematoxylin and eosin (general cytoarchitecture) and Solochrome-cyanine (measurement of corpus callosum, myelination process).
- Immunohistochemistry: GFAP (assessment of astrogliosis), Ki-67 (quantification of mitotically dividing cells), caspase-3 (assessment of the presence of cells undergoing apoptosis), lectin (microcyte reaction).
- Biochemistry: measuring the total capacity of antioxidants present in plasma, measuring glutathione peroxidase present in brain tissue, and measuring malondialdehyde to measure lipid peroxidation.

CHAPTER 4

MATERIALS AND METHODS

This project is in accordance with the Ethical Principles adopted by the Brazilian College of Animal Experimentation (COBEA), protocol no. 114/2012 and approved by the local committee (CETEA - Ribeirão Preto Medical School of USP).

Seven-day-old litters of male Wistar rats from the Bioterium Service of the Ribeirão Preto Administrative Campus are used, in sufficient numbers to make up the experimental groups. Each litter consisted of the mother rat and 8 to 10 pups, which were transported in a single box on the day of birth to the Experimental Surgery Bioterium of the Surgery and Anatomy Department of the Ribeirão Preto Medical School. Fifty rats were needed to carry out all the tests and analyses. Five mother rats were used to care for and breastfeed all the litters (one rat per housing unit), but these rats did not participate directly in the project. During the animals' stay in the vivarium, the standard laboratory diet for rodents and water will be offered *ad libitum* to the mothers. The weaning pups also had access to the diet and water.

4.1. Induction of hydrocephalus

At 7 days of age, the puppies were chosen at random and subjected to induction of hydrocephalus by intracistemal injection of kaolin, under inhalation anaesthesia with isoflurane or kept without intervention to be used as a normal control. To induce hydrocephalus, each animal was positioned by an assistant, who held the head with one hand and the body with the other hand, flexing the animal's neck, leaving the dorsal cervical region free. Palpation identified the space between the posterior margin of the foramen magnum in the occipital bone and the cranial edge of the dorsal arch of the first cervical vertebra (figure 1). A suboccipital puncture was made using a Mise 0.3 dental needle with a short bevel and 0.04ml of a 15% kaolin suspension (Merck®) in distilled water, sterilised in an autoclave, was injected by slow percutaneous injection. The animals were then placed back in their original housing and returned to the vivarium.

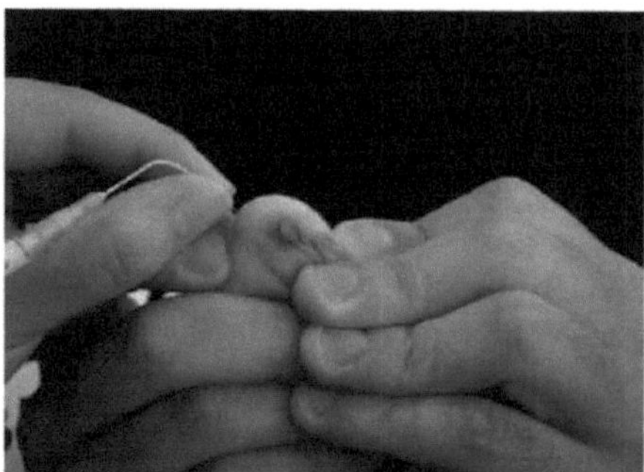

Figure 1 - Induction of hydrocephalus with positioning of the rat by an assistant and percutaneous puncture of the cisterna magna and injection of kaolin by the researcher.

4.2. Formation of the experimental groups

-Control Group (C): Animals sacrificed at 21 days of age (n = 10).

-Hydrocephalus group (HNT): Animals sacrificed 14 days after kaolin injection (21 days old) (n = 20).

-Hydrocephalus Treated Group (HTE): Animals that receive daily intraperitoneal injection of Edaravone (2mg/kg). These animals were sacrificed 14 days after the kaolin injection and treatment (21 days old) (n=20).

All injected animals were observed daily for possible clinical alterations (weight loss and dehydration, changes in gait and consciousness, neglect of hygiene). In the event of the perception of suffering and severe neurological damage, significant weight loss or dehydration that did not respond to hydration with subcutaneous injection of saline solution, the rat was sacrificed with an excessive dose of anaesthetic and was not used in the experiment.

4.3. Behavioural studies

The animals were weighed daily and their general behaviour in the crate was assessed, both individually (exploration of the environment, mobility in space) and in interaction with other members of the group.

To study sensorimotor development, walking behaviour was assessed every 2 days using the open field test *(Open Fiel),* starting on day 6 after injection (P6). Each animal was observed individually in a transparent acrylic arena 60 cm long and 45 cm high. They were timed for 2 minutes and their grooming, environmental exploration and gait were assessed according to the following scale: 4 = alert, with normal exploration and gait; 3 = slightly lethargic, with reduced activity, but normal gait when stimulated; 2 = kyphotic, walks, but gait is broad-based, unstable or ataxic; 1 = can barely walk, but still feeds; 0 = close to death or euthanised. The arena was cleaned with neutral soap diluted in water between observations of different litters of animals.

To study memory and spatial learning, the rats were subjected to the modified Morris *water maze* test. The apparatus consists of a circular pool (100 cm in diameter, 50 cm high) and a transparent platform (34 cm high, 8 cm in diameter) positioned 2 cm below the surface of the water. The pool's water temperature was controlled at approximately 22°C, and it was divided into two phases (adaptation and spatial learning). The adaptation and training phase was carried out on the day corresponding to 9° post-induction of hydrocephalus (P09), during which the rats had 60 seconds free to swim in the pool, without the platform. The platform was then introduced into the tank, positioned in a quadrant (the tank is randomly divided into 4 quadrants). The training was done in four series, each time the animal was placed in the water facing one of the 4 cardinal points. This was done so that the rat would memorise the illuminated wall as a reference point for locating the camouflaged platform under the water surface, rather than randomly finding it by swimming in a straight line. The room housing the tank is completely dark, except for a small light source attached to one of the outer sides of the tank (north), so that the animal can identify the reference point to be memorised. The test was then applied on days P10 and Pll after induction, with the animal being positioned

in each session, facing one of the cardinal points (with 4 sequential sessions), in 2 shifts on the same day. The time limit for the animal to reach the platform and be considered a hit was 60 seconds. At the end of each session, the animal was placed on the platform for a 15-second rest, after which it was returned to the pool wall to start a new session. The time taken from the starting point to the rest platform was timed. The average time for each daily shift was calculated by averaging the time taken to find the platform in each of the 4 sessions. If the animal didn't find the platform by a time limit of 60 seconds, it would be placed on the platform for a 30-second rest, and the time taken to perform the task in that session would be 60 seconds. At the end of the test, the animal was dried off with a soft towel and kept in a warm box, then placed back with its mother and the other pups in the litter. Between each animal examined, all dirt (solid animal waste and particles from the litter) visible in the water of the arena was collected with a sieve.

4.4. Magnetic resonance imaging studies

The animals with hydrocephalus and their controls were taken for magnetic

resonance imaging (MRI) of the brain on the 13th (day) after induction, under anaesthesia with 10% ketamine and 10% intraperitoneal xylazine (at doses of 0.1 and 0.05 mg/lOOg body weight), in a 3T field apparatus, as shown in (figure 2).

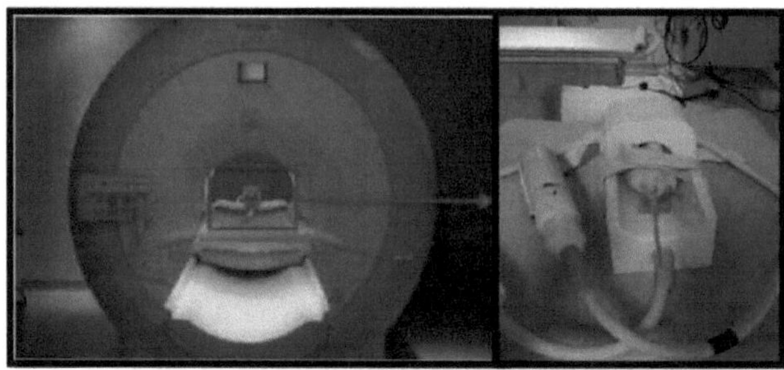

Figure 2- Positioning the animal in the gantry of the 3T MRI scanner, in coil suitable for small rodents, for image acquisition on the 13th day of life.

MR acquisition was carried out on a 3T scanner (Philips, Achieva) using a coil suitable only for small rodents. The protocol included a T2-weighted 3D image and two almost identical MTR/3D sequences (figure 3). The T2 A-weighted 3D sequence was chosen to increase the contrast between cerebrospinal fluid and brain tissue, with high spatial resolution. We used the pre-pulse magnetisation transfer set as the standard "on-resonance" pulse on the Philips MR scanner (consisting of 121 RF pulses with 90° and 4 rectangular elements with a duration of 275 mS each). From both images, the MTR value at each pixel is calculated using the following expression:

MTR [%] = (PiwoMT - PIwMT) - 100 / PiwoMT; where, PIwMT and PiwoMT represent the intensity of the pixels in the image with the pre-pulse magnetisation transfer.

Sequences	3DT2	3DMTR
Echo time	60ms	11ms
Repetition time	1500ms	23ms
Plan	Sagittal	Sagittal
Voxel dimensions	0.3mmx 0.3mm x 0.3mm	0.3mm x 0.3mm x 0.3mm
Thickness	0.3mm	0.3mm

Figure 3 - Details of the sequence parameters.

Manual segmentation of the lateral ventricles and total brain was carried out in the coronal plane in a 3D- T2W image using the STARTX *software for* Linux CYGWIN 4.1.10 *version.* The ventricular ratio (VR) was calculated by dividing the area of the lateral ventricles by the total area of the brain, as follows:

RV = AVL/AVL+AC, where:

LVA = lateral ventricle area (coloured in red in figure 3)

AC = brain area (coloured green in figure 3)

The MTR was also obtained in the mid coronal plane using the whole brain image generated in the segmentation and the MTR map. Magnetisation transfer data was obtained by demarcating areas of interest (ROIs), one in the dorsal region and the other in the ventral region of the lateral ventricle (figure 4).

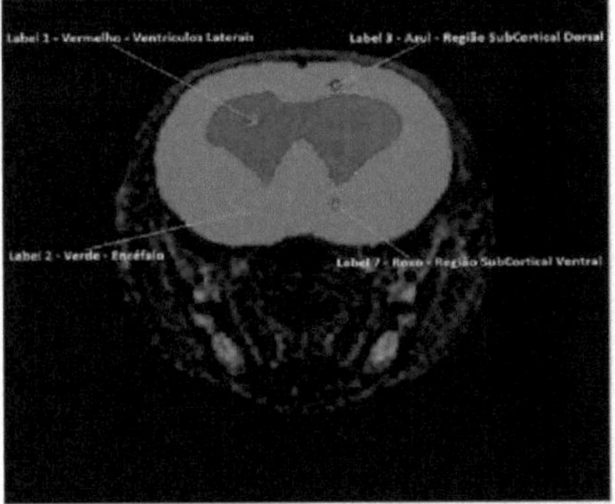

Figure 4- A. MRI image, T2 sequence, medium coronal reconstruction, with delimitation of the areas of interest (ROI) (Blue= dorsal ROI of the lateral ventricle / Violet?ventral ROI of the lateral ventricle) that were used to quantify the myelin, and delimitation of the areas of the encephalon and lateral ventricles to calculate the ventricular ratio (Red area? lateral ventricle / Green area= total encephalon).

4.5. Sample collection: cerebral perfusion and dissection of structures

At the end of the experimental periods, the animals in each group were deeply anaesthetised with intraperitoneal injections of 10% ketamine and 10% xylazine (at doses of 0.1 and 0.05 mg/lOOg body weight). After being positioned on the operating table, in dorsal decubitus, a wide "Y" incision was made in each animal, on the thorax, from the two clavicles to the xiphoid appendix, and on the abdomen, a median, xipho-pubic incision.

In the animals selected for histological and immunohistochemical analysis (half of each group), a 21G needle was inserted into the tip of the left ventricle and cannulated up to the root of the aorta, and transcardiac perfusion with saline solution was started after a small incision in the right auricle, until the outflow fluid was clear (around 1 ml/g of animal weight), using a peristaltic perfusion pump *(Fisher Scientiflc)*. The animals were then decapitated and their brains removed en bloc by means of a craniectomy of the vertex, subdivided in the coronal plane into an anterior and posterior portion, using the optic chiasm as a reference, then immersed in a fixative solution of 3% paraformaldehyde in 0.lM phosphate buffer (pH 7.3 - 7.4) for 24 hours at 4°C, when it was replaced with a fresh 3% paraformaldehyde solution, remaining in this fixative solution for a further 7 days at the same temperature. In the animals selected for biochemical analysis (half of each group), the tip of the left cardiac ventricle was punctured with a 21G needle, introducing it up to the root of the aorta, thus aspirating 2 ml of whole blood and storing it in 1 vacutainer® type vial with heparin, for the dosage of antioxidants present in the plasma, then cardiac perfusion was started. The blood samples were removed and divided in the sagittal plane, frozen in liquid nitrogen and kept in a -80°C freezer for subsequent dosages of total antioxidants, glutathione peroxidase and malondialdehyde.

4.6. Biochemical analysis

The previously frozen brain samples were diluted 1:3 in homogenised buffer using a tissue homogeniser (Polytron - Kinematica PT 1600E). The blood samples, after clot formation, were centrifuged at 2,000 x g at 4°C for 15 min to separate the plasma, which was stored at -80°C. All the samples thus obtained (plasma and tissue) were submitted to biochemical tests using kits, following the manufacturer's instructions.

The "Antioxidant Assay Kit" (Cayman- n°709001) was used to measure the total capacity of antioxidants present in plasma. The previously stored plasma samples were thawed and diluted 1:20 with the appropriate buffer (kit). They were then distributed in duplicate in a 96-well plate alongside the dilutions of the standard. Afterwards, the other reagents in the kit were pipetted in and immediately read at an absorbance of 750 nm according to the manufacturer's instructions.

The "Glutathione Peroxidase Assay Kit (GPx)" (Cayman - n°703102) was used to measure glutathione peroxidase in brain tissue. The samples were thawed and centrifuged at 10,000 g at 4°C for 15 min. Dilutions of the standard solution and the samples were distributed in duplicate in the 96-well plate. Additional reagents from the kit were pipetted in. Gpx activity was calculated from the difference per minute and the plate was read on the reader with an absorbance measurement of 340 nm according to the manufacturer's guidelines.

The "TBARS Assay Kit" (Cayman-n° 1009055) was used to measure malondialdehyde (MDA) (a measure of lipid peroxidation). The previously homogenised brain tissue was thawed and centrifuged at 1,600 g for 10 min at 4°C. The supernatant was cooled and pipetted in duplicates into a 96-well plate, followed by the addition of the kit's other reagents. After the pause time for the chemical reactions, the plate was read in a reader with an absorbance of 530-540 nm according to the manufacturer's guidelines.

4.7. Histochemistry and immunohistochemistry

The brains were dehydrated in increasing amounts of alcohol (50% to 100%), diaphanised in xylene and embedded in paraffin, then cut coronally on a rotary microtome into 5pm-thick sections and the sections spread out on histological slides.

For histochemical analysis, the slides were kept in an oven (60°C) for one hour to melt the paraffin. The sections were then deparaffinised, followed by sequential baths in xylene, alcohol in decreasing concentrations and water; they were then stained with haematoxylin and eosin or solochrome cyanine (each sample was stained with both dyes). The general cytoarchitecture, distribution of structures and cell density were observed (haematoxylin and eosin), while for solochrome-cyanine staining, the degree of myelination of the periventricular white matter was observed and a score of 0 to 2 was applied to assess the blue tone. The greater the shade of blue, the higher the score, and after this process the thickness of the corpus callosum was measured.

For immunohistochemistry, the slides were kept in an oven at 60°C for 30 minutes and deparaffinised in sequential baths of xylene and alcohol. Immunohistochemical studies were carried out for GFAP *(glial fibrillary acidic protein)* to assess the distribution and morphological appearance of astroglia, Ki-67 to assess the germinal matrix in the external angle of the lateral ventricle, capase-3 to assess the presence of damage due to apoptosis and lectin to assess the microcyte reaction. After antigen retrieval, when indicated, using the acidification and heating method (sodium citrate in microwaves), endogenous peroxidase was blocked with 3% hydrogen peroxide in methanol. Subsequently, the endogenous peroxidase was blocked with 10% serum in PBS for 30 minutes in a humid chamber. Afterwards, the sections were incubated *"ovemight"* at 4°C with the primary antibody [anti-GFAP (DAKO Z0334, Denmark), anti-Ki67 (Santa Cruz sc- 23900), anti-caspase-3 (Santa Cruz sc-7148), Lectin (L2140- BS-I sigma)], in appropriate dilutions, previously tested. After removing the primary antibody, the appropriate secondary antibody was added (biotinylated goat anti-rabbit - Santa Cruz Biotechnology SC-2040, or anti-mouse - Santa Cruz Biotechnology SC-2039) diluted 1:300 in BSA (for lectin the secondary antibody is dispensed with). They were then incubated with the HRP-conjugated streptavidin tertiary antibody (BioLegend cat.405210) diluted 1:160 in PBS. They were then stained with DAB (3,3'- diaminobenzidine - Sigma). Finally, the slides were counterstained with haematoxylin, washed in running water, dehydrated in a sequential series of increasing baths of alcohol and xylene, and covered with coverslips mounted with Permount®. Note: for immunohistochemistry, the sections were spread on silanised histological slides.

4.8. Photographic documentation

Photographic documentation of the histological slides was carried out in the Applied and Experimental Neurology laboratory of the Department of Neurosciences and Behavioural Sciences of the Ribeirão Preto Medical School - USP, using an AxiosKop2 plus light microscope (Cari Zeiss) and an AxioCam Hrc digital camera (Cari Zeiss) coupled to a Pentium II computer equipped with Axio Vision 3.1 software, using a 40x objective lens with immersion oil.

For the slides stained with haematoxylin and eosin, the corpus callosum, the germinal matrix, the dorsal cerebral cortex and the external capsule were photographed for later assessment of cytoarchitecture. On the solochrome-cyanine stained slides, the corpus callosum region was photographed to measure its thickness. A visual comparison was also used to apply a score from 0 to 2: 0: weak blue tone; 1: medium blue tone and 2: strong blue tone to assess myelination.

For the GFAP-immunolabelled slides, the corpus callosum and germinal matrix regions were photographed. The images were used to count the reactive astrocytes, and to classify the astroglial reaction, a "score" of 0 to 2 was applied through visual comparison, where 0: no reactive astrocytes; 1: reactive astrocytes with thin, delicate extensions and 2: reactive astrocytes with thick extensions.

For the slides immunolabelled with Ki67, only the region of the germinal matrix at the external angle of the lateral ventricle was photographed (an area of intense cell proliferation), where the immunolabelled cells in mitotic division were counted.

In the slides immunolabelled with caspase-3, the entire length of the corpus callosum and dorsal cerebral cortex was scanned and all the immunolabelled cells in these regions were counted and some of the cells were photographed; for documentation purposes only, the same procedure was carried out on lectin-immunolabelled slides.

The computer programme IMAGEJ version 1.42q, distributed by the National Institutes of Health (NIH), USA, was used to count the cells marked by immunohistochemistry and to measure the thickness of the corpus callosum.

4.9. Statistical analyses

All data are presented as means (x) ± standard error of the mean (SEM). The t-Student test was used to analyse two groups and analysis of variance (ANOVA) was used for three or more groups, followed by Tukey's post-test when indicated for parametric data and Mann-Whitney U test with Dunn's post-test for non-parametric data. Statistical differences are considered when $p<0.05$. A statistical programme for the Windows environment was used, BioEstat version 5.0, developed and distributed by the Mamirauá Sustainable Development Institute, with support from the Ministry of Science and Technology, and for some tests the GraphPadPrismversion 5.0 programme was used (GraphPad Software, Inc. 2007).

CHAPTER 5

RESULTS

5.1. Body weight assessment

All the animals were weighed daily from PO (7 days old) until the end of the experiment on P14 (21 days old). There was no difference in weight between the different experimental groups in the PO.

Group C showed a similar weight gain to the HNT group from the sixth to the eighth day post-induction (P6 to P8) with ($p<0.05$). From P9 onwards, body weight gain was similar in the three experimental groups (figure 5).

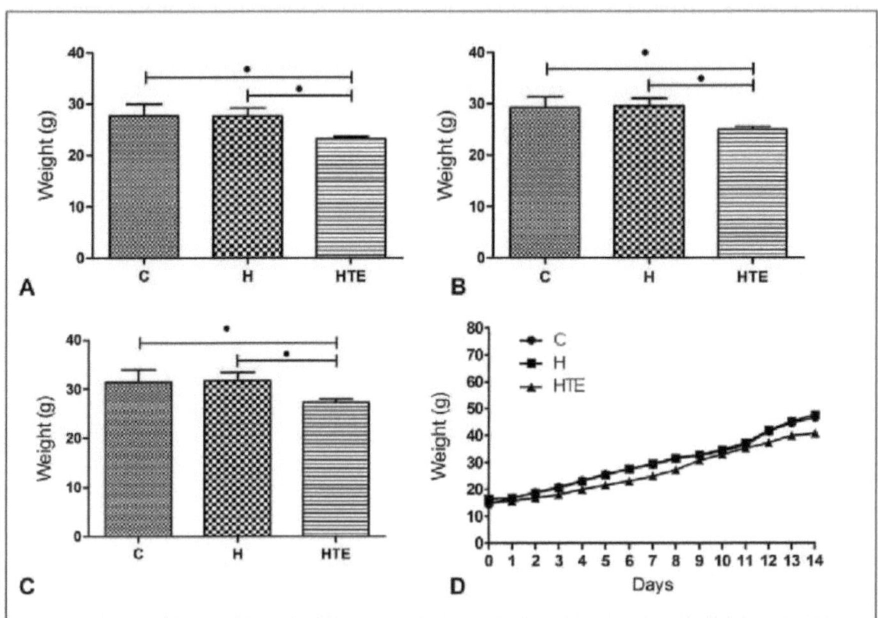

Figure 5- Graph representing the average daily weights of the rats in the different groups experimental. Groups: C: control, H: untreated hydrocephalus and HTE: hydrocephalus treated with edaravone A: P6, B:P7, C:P8, D: evolution of the average daily weights of the animals in the different experimental groups.The control animals (C) showed a similar weight gain to the animals in the HNT group from P6 to P8 ($p<0.05$).

5.2. General behavioural assessment

During the handling of the animals for the daily weighing and cleaning of the box (changing the bedding), the general behaviour of the animals was observed. The HTE group was visibly more active than the untreated hydrocephalic animals, interacting with the environment and exploring it spontaneously. As well as being more attentive, they interacted better with each other, showing more frequent natural behaviours such as fighting and grooming.

5.3. Behavioural assessment with specific tests

5.3.1. Open field test

In the *Open Field* test, carried out on P06, all the experimental groups showed no significant differences. However, on P08, the animals in the HTE group showed better exploration of the environment and a less extended gait pattern when compared to the C and HNT groups, with a statistically significant difference ($p<0.05$). In the IOP test, the animals in the C group showed similar behaviour to the animals in the HTE group, with a static difference when compared to the animals in the HNT group ($p<0.05$). At P12 and P14, the animals in the HTE and C groups showed greater exploration of the environment, normal gait and grooming compared to the animals in the HNT group, with a statistical difference ($p<0.05$) (figure 6).

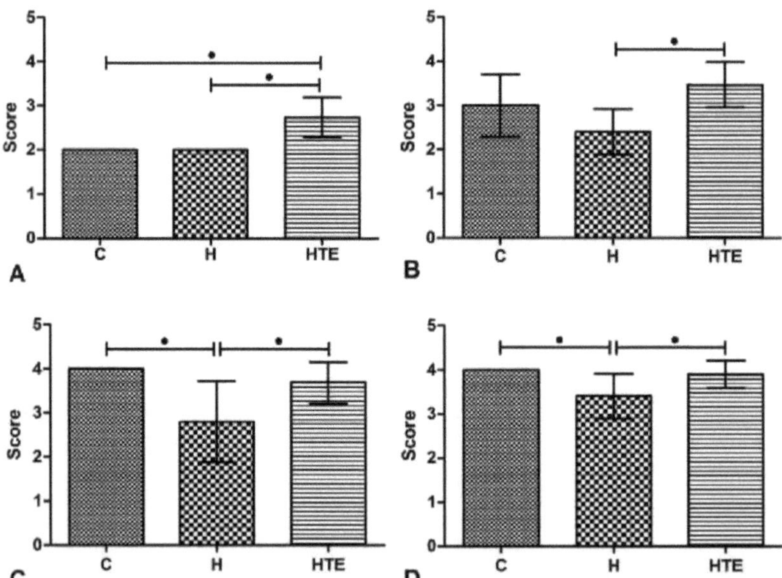

Figure 6: Representative graphs of performance in the open field test. Groups: C: control, H: untreated hydrocephalus and HTE: hydrocephalus treated with edaravone A: P8, B: IOP, C:P12, D: P14. The animals in the HTE group showed greater functional capacity when compared to the other groups ($p<0.05$).

5.3.2 *Water maze*

During the Morris water maze test, carried out in PIO, we can see that, in the morning, the animals in the HTE group had a shorter average time to reach the platform when compared to the animals in the HNT and C groups, with no significant differences. In the afternoon, however, the animals treated with Edaravone performed better and were able to reach the platform with statistically significant differences ($p<0.05$) (C: x=51.60 ± 5.07; HTE: x=45.34 ± 7.80; HNT: x=53.17 ± 8.35). In the Pll during the morning test, the animals in the HNT group had a longer average time than the animals in the HTE and C groups, showing that when performing the test, they took longer to reach the platform, while the animals in the HTE and C groups were learning and memorising the way to reach the platform with a statistical difference ($p< 0.05$), (C: x=34.25 ± 12.40; HTE: x=38.68 ± 13.05; HNT: x=51.60 ± 5.97). In the afternoon, the average time for the three experimental groups was similar (C: x=34.70 ± 12.55; HTE: x=41.36 ± 14.06; HNT: x=43.07 ± 15.46) (figure 7).

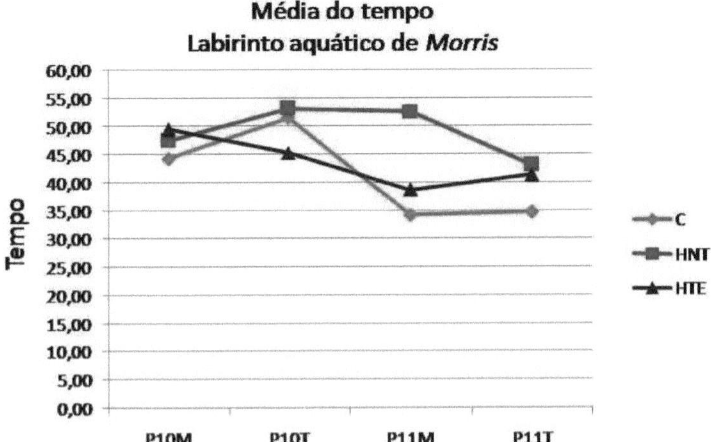

Figure 7: Representative graphs of performance in the memory test (Morris Water Maze), Groups: C: control, HNT: untreated hydrocephalus and HTE: hydrocephalus treated with edaravone showing that the animals in the HTE group performed better (they reached the platform in a shorter time) when compared to the untreated hydrocephalus animals (HNT).

5.4. Magnetic resonance evaluation

5.4.1 Ventricular ratio

Magnetic resonance imaging of the brain quantified the ventricular ratio, calculated from the division (or ratio) between the area of the lateral ventricle in the middle coronal section and the total area of the brain in the same section.

The mean ventricular ratio of the animals in the hydrocephalus groups was similar, with no difference between them, and both showed a higher mean than the animals in the control group with a statistically significant difference ($p<0.01$), (C: x=0.0031 ± 0.0019; HTE: x=0.4432 ± 0.0332; HNT: x=0.5450 ± 0.0581) (figure 8).

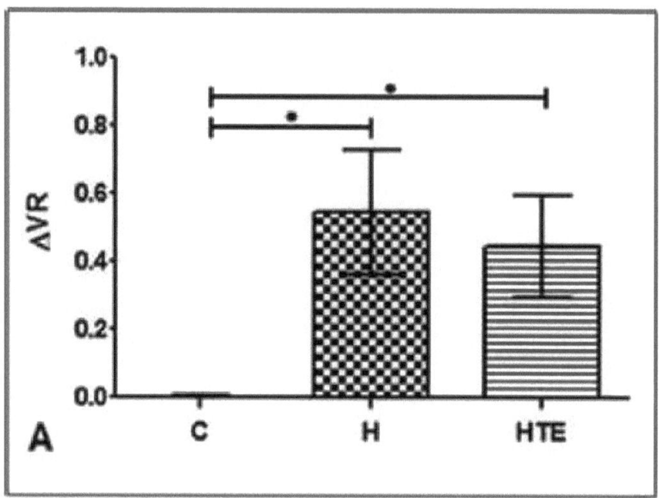

Figure 8 - Graph showing the comparison of ventricular ratio (VR) measurements in the groups studied. Groups: C: control, H: untreated hydrocephalus and HTE: hydrocephalus treated with edaravone. The animals in the HNT/HTE group showed similar VR. When comparing the hydrocephalus groups with group C, the mean VR of both hydrocephalus groups was higher than the mean of the control group ($p<0.01$).

5.4.2 Magnetisation transfer

In the study of magnetisation transfer, in the demarcated regions (dorsal region of the lateral ventricle C: x=28.72 ± 2.21; HTE: x=33.03 ± 2.02; HNT: x=26.7 ± 2.48 and region ventral to the lateral ventricle C: x=44.14 ± 8.28; HTE: x=35.50 ± 1.29; HNT: x=38.97 ± 5.96), no statistically significant differences were observed between the groups investigated. However, when analysing the total brain, the animals in the control group had a higher average number of magnetisation transfers compared to the hydrocephalic animals ($p< 0.05$) (C: x=38.42 ± 4.26; HTE: x=30.27 ± 0.97; HNT: x=32.41 ± 1.87) (figure 9).

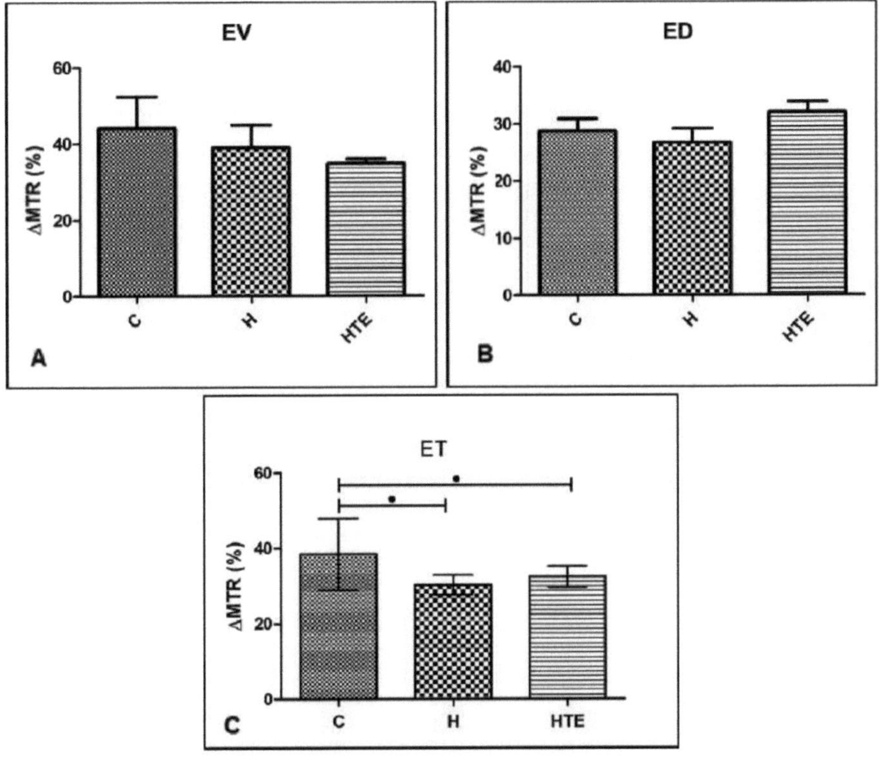

Figure 9 - Representative graph of magnetisation transfer, A: region ventral to the lateral ventricle, B: region dorsal to the lateral ventricle, and C: total encephalon. Groups: C: control, H: untreated hydrocephalus and HTE: hydrocephalus treated with edaravone. There were no differences in the values obtained in the total brain and in the areas dorsal and ventral to the lateral ventricle between the groups studied. In the analysis of the total brain, the control animals had a higher average magnetisation transfer when compared to the animals in the hydrocephalus groups.

5.5. Histochemical evaluations

5.5.1. Haematoxylin and eosin staining

The alterations analysed in the brains of all groups were found especially in the four demarcated regions (corpus callosum, germinal matrix, external capsule, cerebral cortex). The sections with this stain in the control animals showed that the corpus callosum was intact and the ependymal layer covering the lateral ventricles was continuous, with a simple cubic epithelium and ependymal cells with a centralised nucleus. When the general cytoarchitecture was analysed using haematoxylin and eosin staining, the hydrocephalic animals had a larger lateral ventricle with compromised ependyma and flattened cells with rupture points, and the greater the compromise, the greater the ventricular dilation. The corpus callosum was compressed and stretched with signs of oedema, characterised as tears, i.e. lighter areas. In cases of maximum hydrocephalus, the corpus callosum in the midline appears completely destroyed. The dorsal cerebral cortex and external capsule, although compressed and stretched, kept their lamination preserved (figure 10).

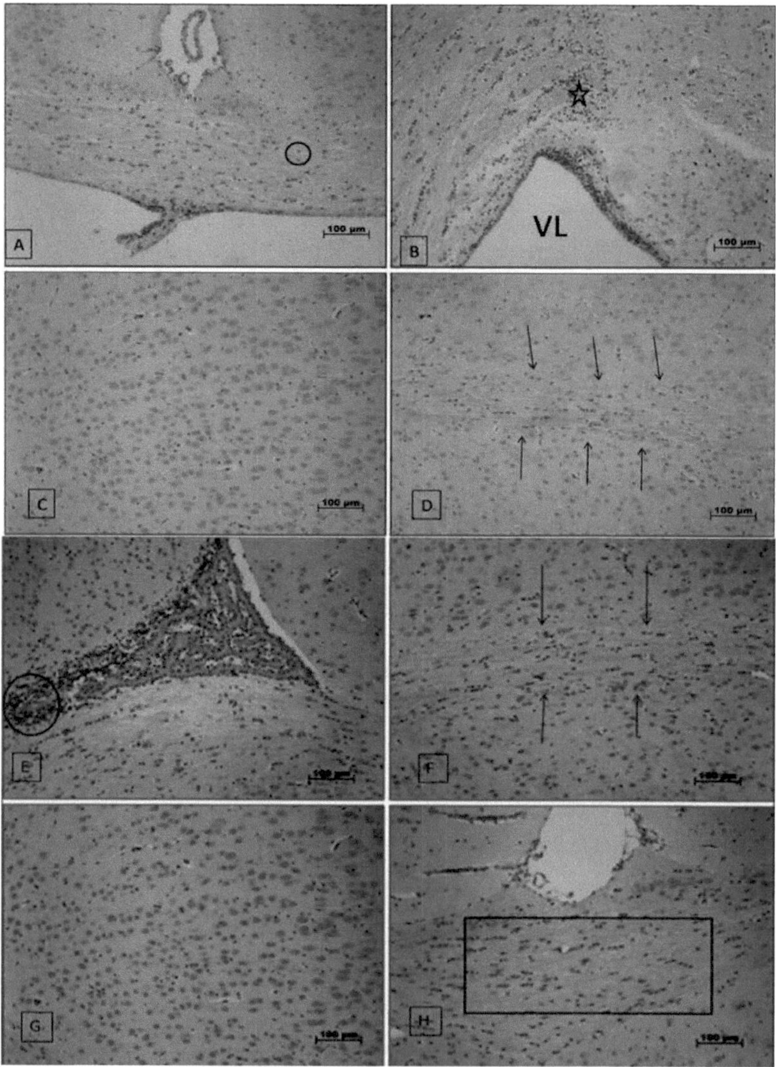

Figure 10 - Photomicrographs of the hydrocephalic rat brain (A) corpus callosum, (B) germinal matrix, (C) cerebral cortex, (D) external capsule (between the arrows), photomicrographs of the control rat brain (E) germinal matrix (F) external capsule (between the arrows), (G) cerebral cortex and (H) corpus callosum (square) (VL) lateral ventricle. Mild oedema (circle), a region of the germinal matrix (star) with a dilated ventricle angle can be seen in the brains of the hydrocephalic rats. In the brains of the control animals, lamination was preserved. Haematoxylin and eosin staining. 40X objective. Bar - lOOpm.

5.5.2. Staining with solochrome-cyanine

In the solochrome-cyanine staining analysis, the degree of myelination of the periventricular white matter, which is stained blue, was assessed through a visual confrontation analysis of the rats' corpus callosum. A *score of* 0 to 2 was applied to classify the intensity of the colouring, with 0 being a weak shade of blue, 1 being a medium shade of blue and 2 being a strong shade of blue (Figure 12). The animals in the control group showed a more intense shade of blue when compared to the hydrocephalus groups (HTEZHNT), indicating a progressive myelination of the corpus callosum, with a statistical difference ($p<0.05$). The comparison of the hydrocephalic animals (HTE and HNT) showed no statistical difference in the mean *score,* but the shade of blue in the corpus callosum of the untreated animals was lighter compared to the group treated with Edaravone. (Figure 11).

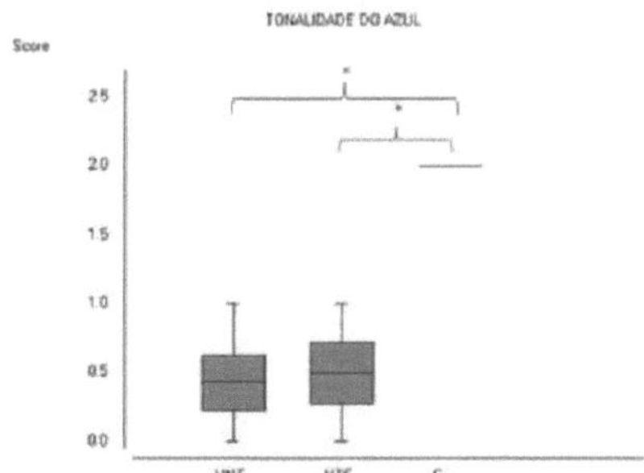

Figure 11 - Comparison of blue tone in the corpus callosum, tabulated using a score from 0 to 2. Groups: C: control, HNT: hydrocephalus without treatment and HTE: hydrocephalus treated with edaravone There was a statistical difference between the hydrocephalus groups compared to the control group, showing that the animals in the control group showed progressive myelination compared to the hydrocephalus animals (*$p<0.05$).

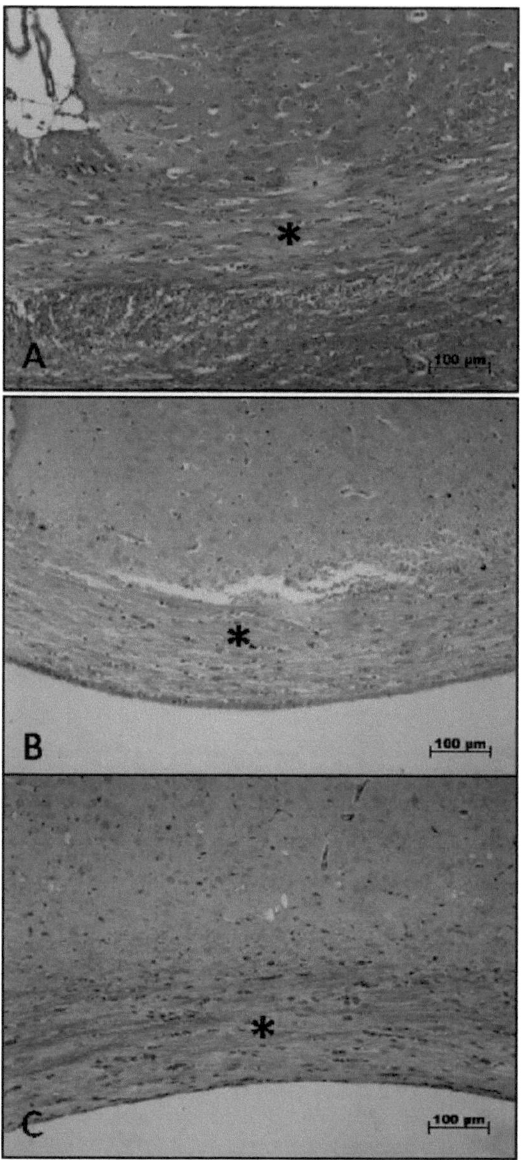

Figure 12 - Photomicrographs of the corpus callosum of rats (21 days old) - (A) Control (B) Untreated hydrocephalus (C) Hydrocephalus treated with Edaravone, showing greater thickness of the corpus callosum in the control animals compared to the hydrocephalus groups. Colour: solochrome-cyanine. 10X objective. Light exposure: 90.0 ms. Bar - 100 pm (*) corpus callosum.

In order to associate the severity of ventriculomegaly with the level of injury, measurements were taken of the thickness of the corpus callosum, which is the structure closest to the lateral ventricles and most susceptible to injury. When comparing the groups (HNT, HTE and C), there was a greater thickness of the corpus callosum in the control animals when compared to both hydrocephalus groups ($p<0.01$). When comparing the HTE and HNT groups, no difference was found (C: $x=214.72 \pm 14.65$; HTE: $x=100.56 \pm 5.68$; HNT: $x=97.91 \pm 2.67$) (figure 13). *Spearman*'s linear correlation coefficient was carried out between corpus callosum thickness and ventricular ratio, showing that there is a correlation between these data with a significant difference ($p<0.0001$) (figure 14).

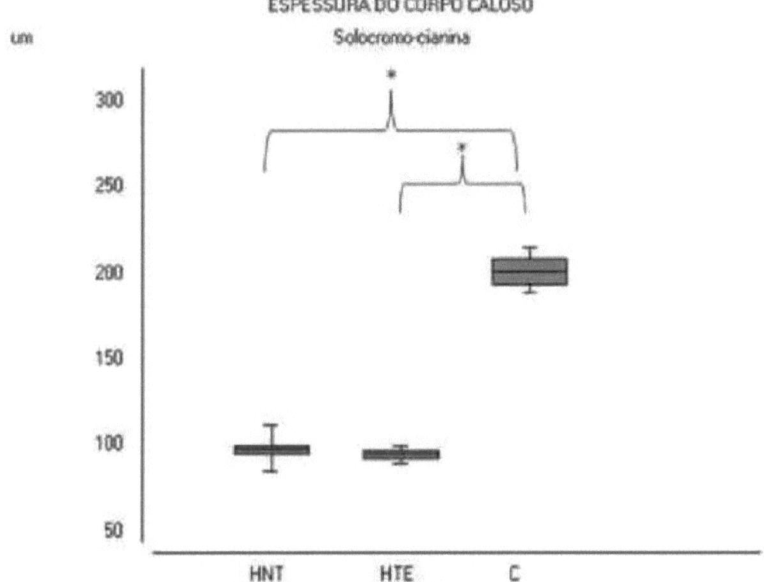

Figure 13 - Comparison of corpus callosum thickness measurements, showing differences between the control and hydrocephalus groups (*$p<0.01$). Groups: C: control, HNT: untreated hydrocephalus and HTE: hydrocephalus treated with edaravone There was no difference between the untreated hydrocephalus group and the group treated with edaravone.

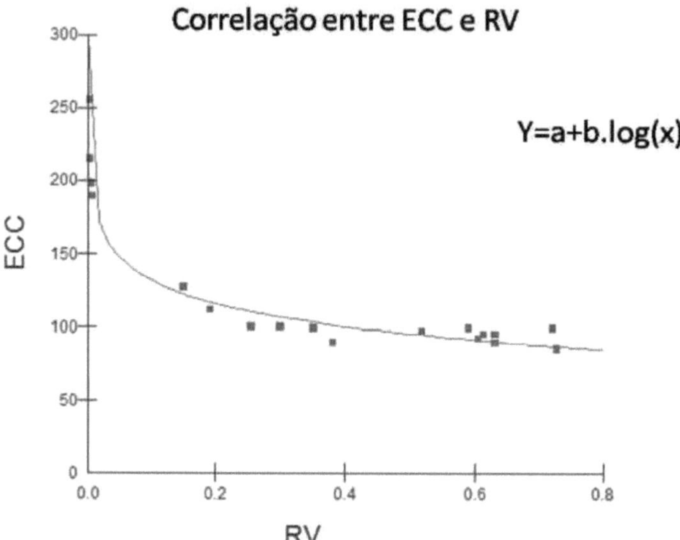

Figure 14 - *Spearman*'s linear correlation ($p<0.0001$). Showing that there is a significant correlation between corpus callosum thickness and ventricular ratio.

5.6. Immunohistochemical evaluations

5.6.1. Immunohistochemical study of GFAP

The astrocytes marked in the corpus callosum and germinal matrix of the animals in the control group showed no signs of hypertrophy, with faint marking and barely visible prolongations. On the other hand, the animals in the HNT group had intensely marked astrocytes with coarser extensions, while the animals treated with Edaravone also had reactive astrocytes, but with finer and more delicate extensions (figure 15). There was a statistical difference when comparing group C with the HNT and HTE groups, with greater astrocyte activity in the hydrocephalic animals ($p<0.05$), for the two regions assessed.

The average number of reactive astrocytes found in the corpus callosum of the different experimental groups were: C: $x=166.67 \pm 72.65$; HNT: $x=1565.0 \pm 412.04$; HTE: $x=2283.33 \pm 1244.51$ and the average number of reactive astrocytes found in the germinal matrix were (C: $x=283.32 \pm 175.89$; HNT: $x=310.83 \pm 169.55$; HTE: $x=380.25 \pm 142.55$) (figure 16).

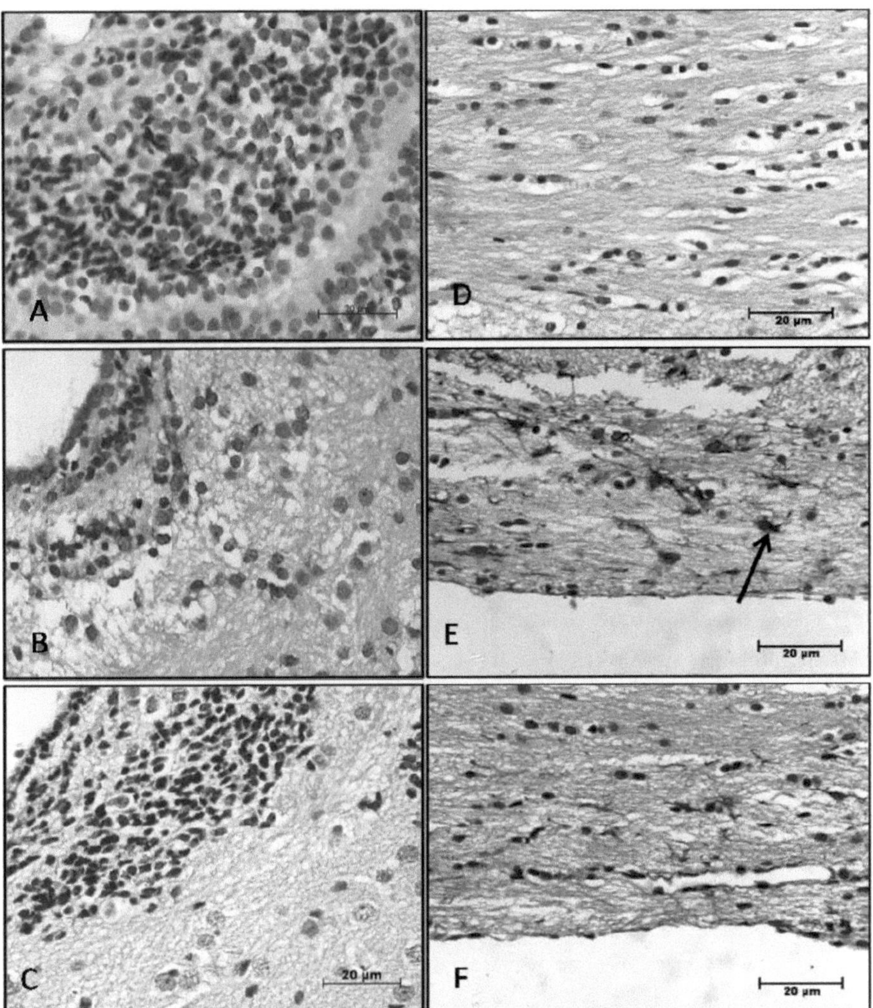

Figure 15 - Photomicrographs of the germinal matrix immunolabelled for GFAP in rats (21 days old) (A) Control (B) Untreated hydrocephalus (C) Hydrocephalus treated with Edaravone. It can be seen that the untreated hydrocephalus group has intensely marked astrocytes when compared to the other experimental groups. Photomicrographs of the corpus callosum immunolabelled for GFAP in rats (21 days old), (D) Control. (E) Untreated hydrocephalus. (F) Hydrocephalus treated with Edaravone. It can be seen that the untreated hydrocephalus group has intensely marked astrocytes when compared to the other experimental groups. 40X objective (immersion). Bar - 20 pm.

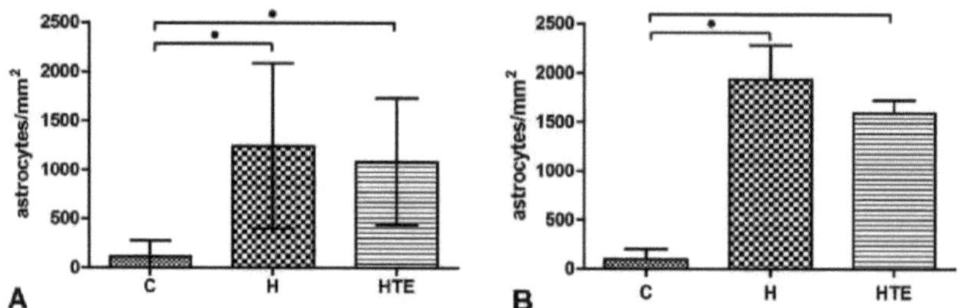

Figure 16 - Representative graph of the density of astrocytes immunolabelled by GFAP. Groups: C: control, H: untreated hydrocephalus and HTE: hydrocephalus treated with edaravone A. in the corpus callosum region and B. germinal matrix in the different experimental groups. Demonstration of animals belonging to the untreated group with a greater astrocyte reaction when compared to the control group *p<0.05.

In classifying astrogliosis using a *score of* 0 to 2, all the photos of the regions studied were observed and tabulated as 0: no reactive astrocytes, 1: reactive astrocytes with thin, delicate extensions and 2: reactive astrocytes with thick extensions. In the areas observed in both the corpus callosum and the germinal matrix, the animals treated with Edaravone showed a lower *score* when compared to the untreated animals, but this difference was not significant. When comparing the HTE/HNT groups with group C, the animals in the control group had a lower mean score than the two hydrocephalus groups (p<0.01) (figure 17).

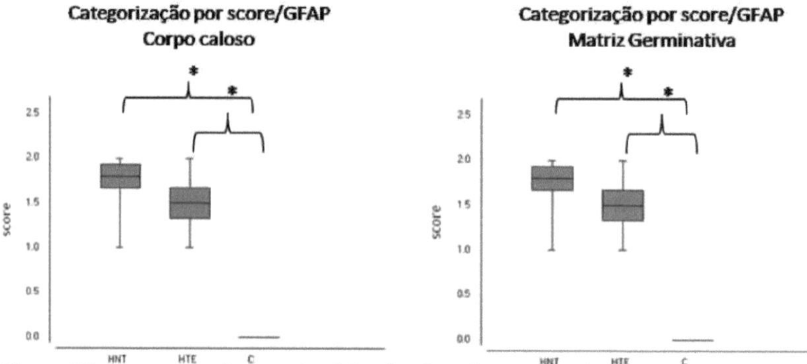

Figure 17 - Representative graph of the density of astrocytes immunolabelled by GFAP categorised by a score. Groups: C: control, HNT: hydrocephalus without treatment and HTE: hydrocephalus treated with edaravone The animals in the HNT group showed more intense and proliferative labelling in the corpus callosum and germinal matrix when compared to the other experimental groups. When comparing the HTE/HNT groups with group C, there was a statistically significant difference, showing that the animals in the control group had a lower mean score than the hydrocephalus groups.

5.6.2. Immunohistochemical study of Ki-67

In the immunohistochemical analysis with Ki-67 antibody, the cells in mitotic division immunolabelled in the region of the germinal matrix, located in the external angle of the lateral ventricles of the brain, were counted.

Comparison of the means between the experimental groups regarding the density of mitotically dividing cells. The comparative analysis of the data from the hydrocephalus groups (HN17HTE) showed no significant difference. However, when comparing the hydrocephalus groups (HNT/HTE) with group C, there was a statistically significant difference; these control animals showed significantly higher cell density in the germinal matrix region than the other groups ($p< 0.01$) (figure 18).

Figure 19 shows the higher density of labelled cells in the germinal matrix of a control rat. In the visual comparison between the untreated and Edaravone-treated hydrocephalus groups, the immunolabelling pattern was similar.

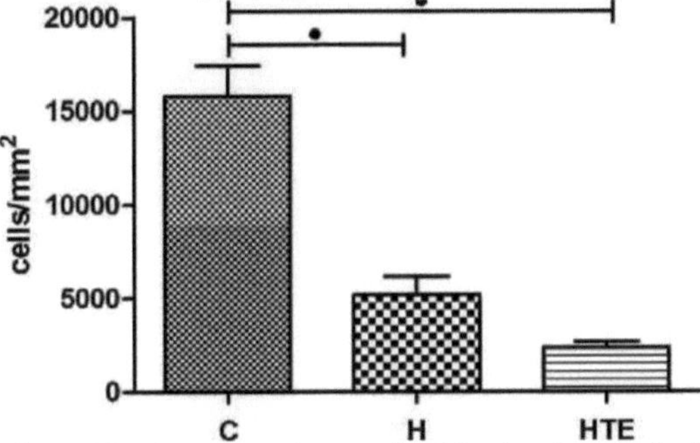

Figure 18 - Representative graph of the density of mitotically dividing cells immunolabelled with the Ki-67 antibody. Groups: C: control, H: untreated hydrocephalus and HTE: hydrocephalus treated with edaravone in the region of the germinal matrix in the different experimental groups. Comparison of the HNTZHTE hydrocephalus groups with group C showed that the animals in the control group had significantly higher cell density than the other groups ($p<0.01$).

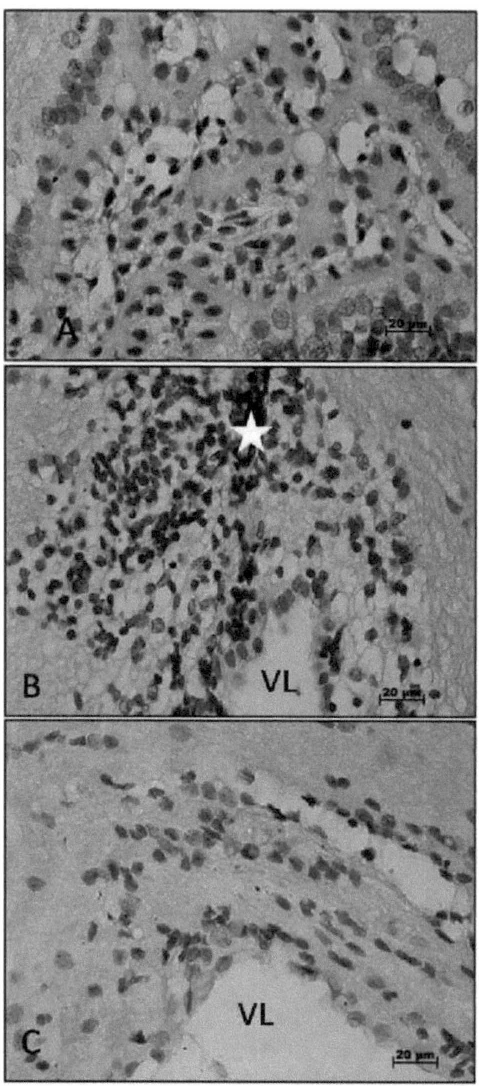

Figure 19 - Photomicrographs of the germinal matrix immunolabelled for Ki-67 in rats (21 days old) (A) Control (B) Untreated hydrocephalus (C) Hydrocephalus treated with Edaravone. It can be seen that group C shows greater cell proliferation when compared to the other experimental groups, cell proliferation (star), lateral ventricle (VL). 40X objective (immersion). Bar - 20 pm.

5.6.3 Caspase-3 immunohistochemical study

In the caspase-3 labelling analysis, the corpus callosum and dorsal cortex regions were scanned and the cells undergoing apoptosis were counted. In the corpus callosum region, there was no statistical difference when comparing the experimental groups, but the animals in the hydrocephalus groups had a higher average number of cells undergoing apoptosis when compared to the control group (C: x=0.22 ±0.11; HTE: x=l.6± 1.24; HNT: x=2.67± 1.65).

In the dorsal cerebral cortex, we observed a statistical difference (p<0.01) (C: x=0.22 ±0.11; HTE: x=l.23± 0.32; HNT: x=l.31± 0.39) between the control group and the HNT group (figure 20).

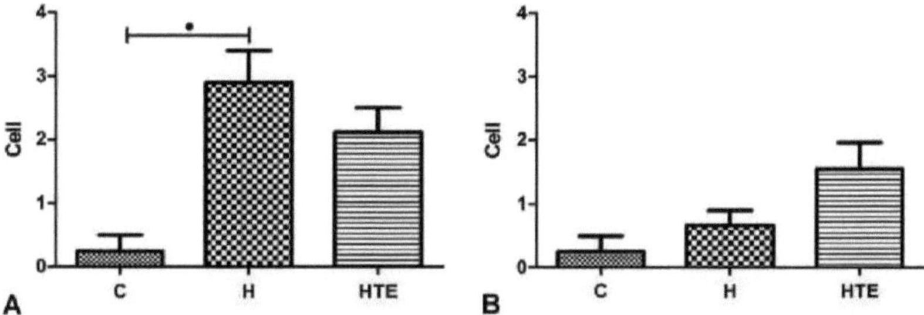

Figure 20 - Representative graph of caspase-3 antibody immunolabelling. Groups: C: control, H: hydrocephalic without treatment and HTE: hydrocephalic treated with edaravone in the (A) dorsal cerebral cortex and (B) corpus callosum, in the different experimental groups (*p<0.01), showing that in the region of the dorsal cortex, the animals in the HTE group had fewer cells undergoing apoptosis compared to the HNT group.

5.6.4 Study of the microglial reaction to lectin

When analysing the slides to study the reaction of microglia cells, no statistical differences were found when comparing the mean counts of marked cells in the dorsal cortex region (cerebral cortex: C: x=0.09 ±0.10; HTE: x=0.91± 0.68;HNT: x=0.95± 1.37). In the corpus callosum, the animals in the HNT group had a higher average when compared to those in the C group (corpus callosum: C: x=0.22 ± 0.33; HTE: x=l.0± 0.61; HNT: x=l.61± 1.13) (figure 21).

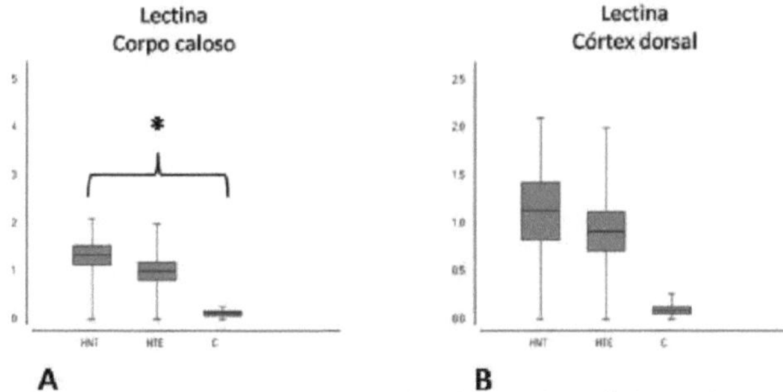

Figure 21 - Representative graph of the microglial reaction. Groups: C: control, HNT: untreated hydrocephalus and HTE: hydrocephalus treated with edaravone (A) corpus callosum and (B) dorsal cortex in the different experimental groups. (A) Shows that the animals in the HNT group had a greater microglial reaction than the animals in group C, with a significant difference (p=< 0.01) in the comparison between the hydrocephalus groups there were no statistical differences.

5.7. Biochemical study

5.7.1 Evaluation of glutathione peroxidase activity

The Glutathione Peroxidase Assay Kit (GPx) was used to measure glutathione peroxidase in brain tissue. By comparing the three experimental groups, no statistically significant differences were found in the means (C: x=0.9 ± 1.02; HTE: x=l.14± 1.24; HNT: x=2.29± 1.87) (Figure 22).

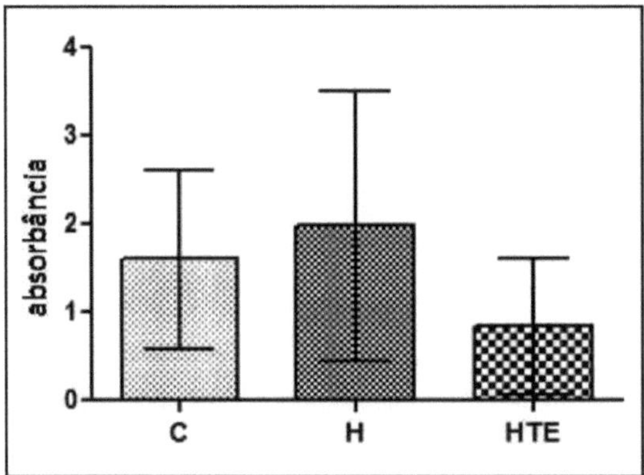

Figure 22 - Representative graph of the glutathione values present in the tissue. Groups: C: control, H: untreated hydrocephalus and HTE: hydrocephalus treated with edaravone. The animals treated with Edaravone showed a lower level of glutathione when compared to the other groups, but without statistical differences.

5.7.2 Evaluation of total antioxidants in plasma

Comparison of the means between the experimental groups showed a statistically significant difference between the hydrocephalus groups in relation to group C, for both HNT and HTE ($p < 0.05$). These animals in the control group had significantly higher amounts of total antioxidants compared to the other groups. However, the comparison of the hydrocephalus groups, HNT and HTE, showed no significant difference (C: x=0.2 ± 0.04; HTE: x=0.08± 0.04; HNT: x=0.10± 0.07) (figure 23).

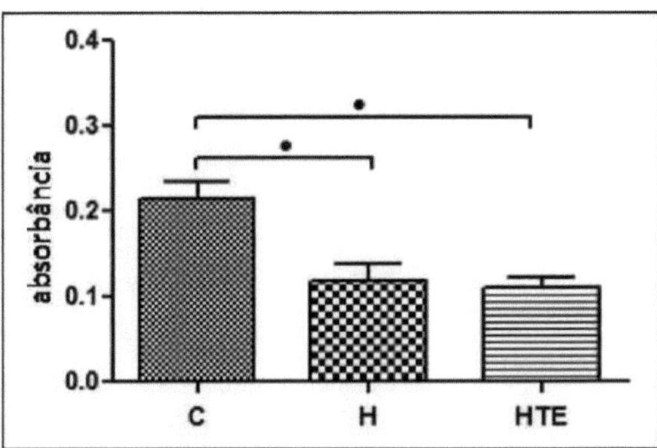

Figure 23 - Representative graph of total antioxidant values in plasma. Groups: C: control, H: untreated hydrocephalus and HTE: hydrocephalus treated with edaravone The animals in group C showed a higher average level of antioxidants when compared to the other groups, with statistically significant differences (*p< 0.05).

5.7.3. Tbars

Lipid peroxidation was assessed by measuring malondialdehyde (MDA) using the TBARS method. No statistically significant differences were found between the 3 groups analysed (C: x=3.5 ± 3.32; HTE: x=6.27± 5.27; HNT: x=6.14± 3.52) (figure 24).

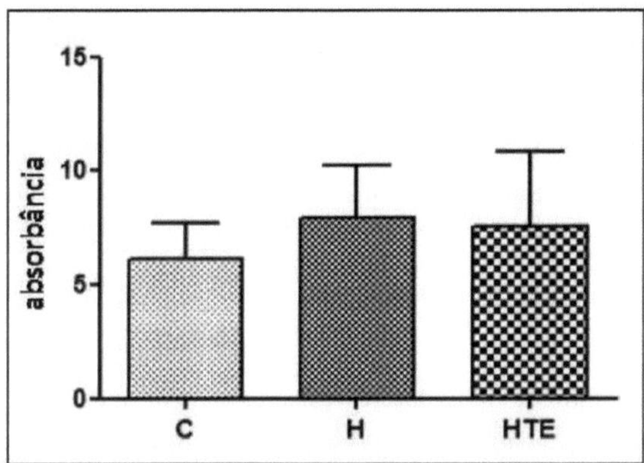

Figure 24 - Representative graph of the malondehyde values present in the tissue. Groups: C: control, H: untreated hydrocephalus and HTE: hydrocephalus treated with edaravone The animals treated with edaravone showed a higher level when compared to the other groups, but without statistical differences.

CHAPTER 6

DISCUSSION

The purpose of this study was to evaluate the role of free radical production in the encephalic lesions found in experimental hydrocephalus induced in young rats, and to test a drug with an antioxidant effect, Edaravone, which has never been used in the treatment of hydrocephalus. The evaluation considered data obtained through the evolution of the animals' daily weight gain, behavioural analysis with specific tests to assess learning capacity, memory and sensorimotor development, histopathological studies to ascertain the general cytoarchitecture and myelination of the encephalon, immunohistochemical analyses to determine the degree of astrogliosis, the number of mitotically dividing cells in the germinal matrix and cell death by apoptosis, biochemical studies with dosages of total antioxidants in the blood and measurement of lipid peroxidation in the nervous tissue.

Evaluating weight gain provides relevant data in relation to the progression of the disease and the level of dehydration of the animals with hydrocephalus. Our results showed no significant difference in the mean weights between the 3 experimental groups studied, but between P6 and P8, group C showed a greater weight gain when compared to the hydrocephalus groups (HNT, HTE). When comparing HNT and HTE, the animals in the HTE group gained less weight than the animals in the HNT group. This could be explained by the fact that the animals in the HTE group, as well as suffering the stress of hydrocephalus, also received a daily intraperitoneal injection of the drug tested, which could lead to inhibition of the search for food due to pain. From P9 onwards, the animals in all groups showed similar weight gain. This finding could be the result of adaptation to the pathological condition. Catalão *et al.* found similar results of body weight variation in kaolin-induced hydrocephalus in Wistar rats, i.e. in the first half of the experiment, the animals with hydrocephalus gained less weight than the controls, but this difference decreased until, at the end of the experiment, the untreated hydrocephalic animals showed weight gain similar to that of the healthy controls (CATALAO *et al.,* 2014).

Measuring the animals' locomotor activity in open field tests can be useful for evaluating the progression of the disease and the effectiveness of the treatments instituted. In general, the open field test has the advantage of being easy to perform, with no need to handle the animal during the test, as it is non-invasive and can be performed several times during the experimental period (TATEM *et al.,* 2014). However, it *is* a semi-quantitative test, as a *score* is assigned to each animal's performance, *which* may include an error of judgement on the part of the observer. In order to assess motor and exploratory activity, the animals were subjected to the open field test on experimental days P06, P08, PIO, P12 AND P14. On P06, the animals from the different experimental groups, including the controls, showed difficulty in gait execution, presenting a dorsal kyphotic curvature, an unbalanced gait and a widened base. These signs are considered standard in rats of this age, as the animal's brain has not completed its development and maturation (TATEM *et al.,* 2014). At P8 the animals in the Edaravone-treated group showed greater exploration in the arena, a less extended gait pattern, quantity of fighting movements and body cleaning, with a statistically significant difference when compared to those in the HNT and C groups. In the IOP test, the animals in group C showed similar behaviour to the animals in the HTE group, with a statistical difference when compared to the animals in the HNT group. As for PI2 and P14, the animals in the HTE and C groups showed greater environmental exploration, normal gait and hygiene care compared to the animals in the HNT group. These results may indicate that the animals treated with Edaravone improve their motor activity. However, signs of fighting and excessive grooming may indicate that the animals are experiencing an increased level of irritability, which could be a result of the daily injection of the drug tested.

In the modified Morris water maze test, the animals in the different groups were trained to find a submerged platform in a dark room, using a faint light source on the north wall of the room that housed the tank as a reference. This training was done in four series, each time the animal was placed in the water facing one of the four cardinal points. This was done so that the rat would memorise the illuminated wall as a reference point for locating the camouflaged platform under the water surface, rather than randomly finding it by swimming in a straight line. To assess the ability to memorise the location of the platform, each animal was assessed on PIO and Pll days, in 4 sets in the morning and 4 sets in the afternoon (one at each cardinal point). The swimming time was timed from the moment the animal was placed in the water until it climbed onto the platform. After reaching the platform, the animal was given 15 seconds to rest on it. If the rat didn't find the platform within 60 seconds, this time was considered the timing and the animal was placed on the platform for 15 seconds. Other groups of researchers have used the same type of test to assess performance in learning and memorising a referenced water route to a submerged platform in experimental hydrocephalus in rats (DEL BIGIO; WILSON; ENNO, 2003, HU *et al.,* 2014). In the morning assessment of the IOP day, the animals from the different experimental groups had a similar average time to find the platform. In the afternoon session at PIO and the morning session at PH, the animals treated with Edaravone had a shorter average time to reach the submerged platform. However, in the afternoon session on day PI 1, the 3 experimental groups performed the test with similar average times. These results may show that the animals in the HTE and C groups learned and memorised the way to reach the platform more quickly than the hydrocephalic animals that did not receive treatment (HNT), showing a tendency towards encephalic maturation. However, histopathologically, no results were found regarding maturation. Future studies would require tests to understand the action of Edaravone on the memorisation of hydrocephalic rats and analyses of synaptic connectivity and neuronal metabolism to better explain these findings.

Magnetic resonance imaging of the brain quantified the ventricular ratio, calculated from the division (or ratio) between the area of the lateral ventricle in the medial coronal section and the total area of the brain in the same section. The hydrocephalic rats in the HTE and HNT groups had ventriculomegaly of varying degrees. The magnetic resonance images corresponded to the images seen later on histology, with an increase in both the lateral and vertical diameters of the lateral ventricles. The mean ventricular ratios of the animals in the hydrocephalus groups were similar to each other, and both groups had significantly higher means than the animals in the control group. The ventricular ratio showed a very large variance in the two hydrocephalus groups, indicating the varying degrees of ventriculomegaly in these animals. The degree of ventriculomegaly is a factor that we were unable to control, as the animals show an inflammatory reaction to the kaolin injection at the exit of the fourth ventricle, of varying intensity, which may be related to the particular conditions of each rat. Different MRI techniques have been used in hydrocephalus studies to quantify myelin and assess the concentration of metabolites resulting from tissue degradation (YAMADA *et al.*, 1992, BRAUN *et al.*, 1997, CORKILL *et al.*, 2003, YUAN *et al.*, 2009, CASTRO *et al.*, 2012). Magnetisation transfer (MTR) is an MRI technique that has been used to quantify the myelin present in different areas of the brain, but had not yet been used by other groups in studies of experimental hydrocephalus. This analysis is based on the exchange of magnetisation between protons, which are bound to large molecules with low mobility, such as myelin, and mobile protons in free water (GOZZI *et al.,* 2012). Quantification of the MTR rate is used to investigate the degree of destruction of central nervous system tissue in humans and animals, since reductions in MTR values are attributed to a decrease in the integrity of macromolecules, reflecting damage to myelin (NEWBOULD *et al.,* 2014), the axonal membrane, or dilution of macromolecules in inflammatory oedema (ZAARAOUI *et al.,* 2008). In a previous hydrocephalus study carried out by our group, MTR was shown to be related to periventricular white matter damage, with reduced values compared to normal controls. When hydrocephalic rats were treated with cerebrospinal fluid shunts and these were functional, MTR values returned to those obtained in the brains of normal rats (ROCHA CATALAO *et al.,* 2014). Our results show that when analysing the total brain, the animals in the control group had slightly higher MTR values than the hydrocephalic animals.

Histological analysis using H&E staining assessed the general cytoarchitecture in different brain regions (germinal matrix, external capsule, cerebral cortex, corpus callosum, hippocampus). The brains of the animals belonging to group C showed preserved cortical lamination, with no anatomical alterations. The hydrocephalic animals showed markedly enlarged lateral ventricles and, in cases of more severe hydrocephalus, the third ventricle was also dilated. The corpus callosum in these animals was compressed and stretched, with signs of oedema such as fraying and less stained areas between the nerve fibres, while the dorsal cerebral cortex, although compressed, maintained its lamination. It was possible to identify the loss of integrity of the ependyma, which showed flattened cells with rupture points, and this impairment increased with the level of ventricular dilation. In cases of maximum hydrocephalus, the midline of the brain was sometimes completely destroyed. There were no obvious differences between the group treated with Edaravone and the untreated hydrocephalus group. Therefore, we believe that the histopathological analysis alone was not sufficient to demonstrate alterations in the structures that would have been reversed with the use of Edaravone at the doses and experimental times studied.

In 1997, Del Bigio and colleagues used the same method to assess the degree of myelination and obtained positive results in terms of the reliability of the analysis (DEL BIGIO; KANFER; ZHANG, 1997). In our analysis, solochrome-cyanine staining was used to assess the degree of myelination of the periventricular white matter,

stained blue by the method. As the intensity of the blue is directly proportional to the degree of myelination, it was possible to relate the hydrocephalus lesion to the loss of myelin and assess whether the drug tested had any effect on myelination. The animals in the control group showed a significantly more intense blue colour in the corpus callosum when compared to the hydrocephalus groups (HTE and HNT). When we compared the corpus callosum of the animals in the two hydrocephalus groups, we could see that the intensity of the blue colouring seemed more intense in the rats treated with Edaravone, suggesting a better myelination pattern in this region, which could be the result of the neuroprotective effect of the drug. However, when we assigned a blue colour intensity *score*, making this assessment less subjective, we observed no significant difference between the treated and untreated hydrocephalic animals.

To associate the degree of ventriculomegaly with the severity of damage to the corpus callosum (the structure closest to the cavities of the lateral ventricles), measurements were taken of its thickness. When comparing the groups (HNT, HTE and C), there was a greater thickness of the corpus callosum in the control animals, with a statistically significant difference. In the comparison between the HTE and HNT groups, no significant difference was found. The purpose of our study was not to use Edaravone to prevent the progression of ventricular dilation, but rather to attenuate the lesions in the brain parenchyma resulting from the generation of free radicals.

Astrocytes are neuroglia cells widely distributed throughout the central nervous system, both in the white and grey matter. They perform important functions, such as supporting and nourishing neurons, as well as regulating neuronal functions. Astrocytes are activated in situations of aggression against the central nervous system, in a defensive response, limiting and repairing tissue damage and restoring homeostasis. One of the characteristics observed during glial activation is the increased expression of GFAP, in a process called reactive astrogliosis, which occurs in situations such as trauma, genetic disorders, chemical insults and neurodegenerative diseases (PEKNY; PEKNA, 2014). Our results from the histopathological analysis using immunohistochemistry for GFAP showed that the immunolabelled astrocytes in the different regions studied in the rats with untreated hydrocephalus were intensely marked and had thick extensions. On the other hand, in the hydrocephalic animals treated with Edaravone, the astrocytes were more delicate with thinner extensions, although we observed more intense astrocyte immunolabelling than in the control rats. This coarser appearance of the astrocytes is precisely because these cells are activated to repair and heal the central nervous system in the most different types of aggression. However, in addition to the qualitative analysis, we counted and calculated the density of reactive astrocytes in the corpus callosum and germinal matrix, areas chosen because they showed the most obvious astrogliosis. Our results showed no significant difference in astrocyte density in these regions between the HTE and HNT hydrocephalus groups. These findings suggest that Edaravone may have played a minimal neuroprotective role when considering the intensity of the astrocyte reaction, but the number of immunolabelled astrocytes was similar in both groups. In other models of nerve tissue damage, such as cerebral ischaemia and traumatic brain injury, Edaravone has been shown to be effective in reducing lesions by acting on biomolecular mechanisms related to oxidative stress (WANG *et al.*, 2011, REN *et al.*, 2014). The fact that we found only a slight improvement in brain lesions may mean that oxidative stress may not represent a very important mechanism in the genesis of these lesions and, therefore, a drug with antioxidant action does not play a relevant role in neuroprotection.

When analysing cells in mitotic division immunolabelled by Ki-67, we examined the region of the germinal matrix (located at the external angle of the lateral ventricles of the brain, a region of intense cell proliferation), which is still present in young rats. We observed that the animals in the control group showed intense cellularity in this region, with a large number of cells immunolabelled by Ki-67. On the other hand, the hydrocephalic animals, both treated and untreated with Edaravone, showed less obvious immunolabelling, with reduced cellularity in the region studied and, after counting the immunolabelled cells, we observed no significant difference between these two hydrocephalic groups. We can therefore conclude that Edaravone, at the dose tested and during the experimental observation period, was not sufficient to protect the germinal matrix region. In a study of hydrocephalic animals treated with quercetin, a drug with great antioxidant action, a marked increase in cell proliferation was observed, analysed by immunolabelling for Ki-67 in the cells of the walls of the lateral ventricles. The authors state that the accumulation of reactive oxygen species impairs the proliferation and self-renewal of neural stem cells, and the antioxidant tested may act by co-operating in restoring homeostasis and preventing cell damage (LI, X. *et al.,* 2014). The fact that we did not observe a recovery in cellularity in the germinal matrix region with the use of Edaravone may indicate that the dose of the drug we used was not sufficient to obtain the beneficial effects.

In the caspase-3 labelling analysis, the regions of the corpus callosum and cerebral cortex dorsal to the corpus callosum were studied. By scanning these areas, we counted all the immunolabelled cells (in the process of apoptosis). We observed no difference in the count of cells marked by caspase-3 in the corpus callosum between the three groups analysed. On the other hand, in the dorsal cortex, we observed that the HNT group had a higher number of cells undergoing apoptosis when compared to the HTE and C groups. These results suggest a beneficial effect of Edaravone in hydrocephalic animals, as it reduces cell death by apoptosis in the cerebral cortex. Some authors have already suggested that Edaravone, in addition to its antioxidant effect in cerebral ischaemia, plays a relevant role in reducing apoptosis and consequent cell death (LI, Q. *et al.*, 2014). As we found a difference in the count of cells in apoptosis immunolabelled by caspase-3 only in the cerebral cortex dorsal to the corpus callosum, but not in the corpus callosum itself, we can deduce that these brain-dead cells are neurons. However, double-labelled immunohistochemistry will be necessary to confirm this.

Microglia correspond to the group of immune system cells in the central nervous system and play a crucial role, both physiologically and in pathological conditions, such as restoring the integrity of the central nervous system and slowing down the progression of neurodegenerative diseases. The physiological role of microglia in brain development is still largely unknown. It is known that during development it is capable of phagocytising and acting in the regulation of apoptosis, cell proliferation, neuronal differentiation and angiogenesis. It may also have a dual function as a mediator of inflammation and aid in the recovery process after damage to the central nervous system (CZEH; GRESSENS; KAINDL, 2011). In our results regarding the evaluation of the reaction of microglia cells through lectin labelling, we found no difference in the count of these cells in the cerebral cortex dorsal to the corpus callosum between the 3 groups studied. However, in the corpus callosum, the animals in the HNT group had a significantly higher average number of cells with microglial reaction when compared to the rats in the C group. On the other hand, the mean count of lectin-labelled cells in the corpus callosum of the HTE group was not statistically different when compared to both the HNT group and the control group. With ventriculomegaly, the corpus callosum is the most damaged structure, as it is one of the closest to the lateral ventricles, thus having more action from the microglia cells. The beneficial effect of Edaravone seems to have been only slight, as the number of cells labelled by the lectin in the corpus callosum of the rats in the HTE was between the counts of the control and HNT groups, but there was no significant difference.

Several oxygen free radicals, including superoxide, hydroxyl radical, nitric oxide and hydrogen peroxide, have been implicated in the development of various neurological disorders and brain dysfunctions (SIESJO; AGARDH; BENGTSSON, 1989, CHAN, 1994). These radicals are known to initiate lipid peroxidation and cause protein oxidation and cell DNA damage. Diseases with global cerebral ischaemia damage are related to oxidative stress caused by excessive production of EROS and other free radicals (NISHINO; TAMURA, 1991). Enzymatic and non-enzymatic mechanisms are the central nervous system's defence against oxidative stress. When there is no effective "scavenging" by the antioxidant systems, free radicals begin to accumulate and damage the tissue. Studies suggest that oxidative damage to the brain may be an important factor in the pathogenesis of hydrocephalus (DI CURZIO; TURNER- BRANNEN; DEL BIGIO, 2014, LI, X. *et al.,* 2014). Other researchers also suggest that Edaravone is a great antioxidant agent, which inhibits the generation of free radicals, thus preventing cell death induced by oxidative stress (SHOKRZADEH *et al.*, 2014, TSURUOKA *et al.,* 2014).

In an attempt to associate the use of Edaravone with neuroprotection in hydrocephalus, we measured the total antioxidants present in plasma, quantified lipid peroxidation and the activity of an enzyme involved in the process of regulating the production of free radicals in brain tissue.

No difference was observed between the two hydrocephalus groups in the quantification of total antioxidants in plasma. On the other hand, the control group had significantly more antioxidants in its plasma than the two groups of rats with hydrocephalus. Glutathione peroxidase is an endogenous antioxidant enzyme found in all animal cells. Its level is reduced in the presence of free radicals and oxidative stress, as it is used to regulate and cleanse these products. In this study, this enzyme was measured in brain tissue and its consumption over time was taken into account. No significant differences were found between the means of the three experimental groups.

Lipid peroxidation products are known to increase immediately after tissue damage. MDA is formed from the breakdown of polyunsaturated fatty acids and serves as a convenient indicator for determining the extent of lipid peroxidation. To assess malondialdehyde levels, we used the measurement of thiobarbituric acid reactive substances. We also found no significant differences in the average MDA level between the 3 groups analysed. The fact that we didn't find antioxidant levels that could suggest the beneficial action of Edaravone could mean that the dose we used may not have been enough to increase the amount of antioxidants in the plasma and tissue, since we didn't do a dose-dependence study. Similarly, another study using a set of antioxidant drugs showed that hydrocephalus-treated animals did not obtain an increase in MDA levels (DI CURZIO; TURNER-BRANNEN; DEL BIGIO, 2014).

At the dose tested, Edaravone did not show a relevant antioxidant effect, although we did observe a beneficial role in cell death by apoptosis. Therefore, other doses of the drug deserve to be tested. On the other hand, we know that cerebral ischaemia is one of the mechanisms of tissue damage in hydrocephalus, occurring due to compression and distortion of the cerebral vessels, especially the smaller calibre vessels, and the presence of high levels of free radicals in hydrocephalus may be associated with reperfusion following *shunt* placement for its treatment. Therefore, further studies should be carried out associating the treatment of hydrocephalus with cerebrospinal fluid shunting and the use of Edaravone.

CHAPTER 7

CONCLUSIONS

1. The animals treated with Edaravone were more active, with greater performance in exploring the environment and better sensorimotor development, learning and memorisation.
2. Histological evaluation using solochrome-cyanine proves the detrimental role that hydrocephalus plays on the myelination of structures.
3. Edaravone administered for 14 consecutive days from the induction of hydrocephalus reduced astrocyte activity as evidenced by GFAP immunolabelling in the corpus callosum and germinal matrix.
4. Progressive ventricular dilatation in hydrocephalus contributes to the disappearance of migratory cells in the germinal matrix region, as evidenced by Ki67 immunolabelling.
5. Edaravone did not show antioxidant activity at the doses tested, but it did show a neuroprotective action against cell death by apoptosis and a decrease in the microglial reaction of the corpus callosum.
6. At the dose tested, Edaravone did not show an increase in total antioxidant levels, requiring studies with other doses.

CHAPTER 8

REFERENCES

ATES, O.; CAYLI, S.; ALTINOZ, E.; GURSES, L; YUCEL, N.; SENER, M.; KOCAK, A.; YOLOGLU, S. Neuroprotection by resveratrol against traumatic brain injury in rats. **Mol Cell Biochem,** v. 294, n. 1-2, Jan, p.137-144. 2007.

BANNO, M.; MIZUNO, T.; KATO, H.; ZHANG, G.; KAWANOKUCHI, J.; WANG, J.; KUNO, R.; JIN, S.; TAKEUCHI, H.; SUZUMURA, A. The radical scavenger Edaravone prevents oxidative neurotoxicity induced by peroxynitrite and activated microglia. **Neuropharmacology,** v. 48, n. 2, Feb, p.283-290. 2005.

BONDURANT, C. P.; JIMENEZ, D. F. Epidemiology of cerebrospinal fluid shunting. **Pediatr Neurosurg,** v. 23, n. 5, p.254-258; discussion 259. 1995.

BRAUN, K. P.; DE GRAAF, R. A.; VANDERTOP, W. P.; GOOSKENS, R. H.; TULLEKEN, K. A.; NICOLAY, K. In vivo 1H MR spectroscopic imaging and diffusion weighted MRI in experimental hydrocephalus. **Magn Reson Med,** v. 40, n. 6, Dec, p.832- 839.1998.

BRAUN, K. P.; DUKHUIZEN, R. M.; DE GRAAF, R. A.; NICOLAY, K.; VANDERTOP, W. P.; GOOSKENS, R. H.; TULLEKEN, K. A. Cerebral ischaemia and white matter oedema in experimental hydrocephalus: a combined in vivo MRI and MRS study. **Brain Res,** v. 757, n. 2, May 23, p.295-298. 1997.

CANER, H.; ATASEVER, A.; KILINC, K.; DURGUN, B.; PEKER, S.; OZCAN, O. E. Lipid peroxide levei increase in experimental hydrocephalus. **Acta Neurochir (Wien),** v. 121, n. 1- 2, p.68-71. 1993.

CASTRO-GAGO, M.; RODRIGUEZ, I. N.; RODRIGUEZ-NUNEZ, A.; GUITIAN, J. P.; ROCAMONDE, S. L.; RODRIGUEZ-SEGADE, S. Therapeutic criteria in hydrocephalic children. **Childs Nerv Syst,** v. 5, n. 6, Dec, p.361-363. 1989.

CASTRO, S. C.; MACHADO, H. R.; CATALAO, C. H.; SIQUEIRA, B. A.; SIMÕES, A. L.; LACHAT, J. J.; LOPES LDA, S. 0.1T magnetic resonance imaging in the study of experimental hydrocephalus in rats. Accuracy of the method in the measurements of the ventricular size. **Acta Cir Bras,** v. 27, n. 11, Nov, p.768-772. 2012.

CATALAO, C. H.; CORRÊA, D. A.; SAITO, S. T.; LOPES LDA, S. Camellia sinensis neuroprotective role in experimentally induced hydrocephalus in Wistar rats. **Childs Nerv Syst,** v. 30, n. 4, Apr, p.591-597. 2014.

CHAN, P. H. Oxygen radicals in focal cerebral ischaemia. **Brain Pathol,** v. 4, n. 1, Jan, p.59-65.1994.

CORKILL, R. G.; GARNETT, M. R.; BLAMIRE, A. M.; RAJAGOPALAN, B.; CADOUX-HUDSON, T. A.; STYLES, P. Multi-modal MRI in normal pressure hydrocephalus identifies pre-operative haemodynamic and diffusion coefficient changes in normal appearing white matter correlating with surgical outcome. **Clin Neurol Neurosurg,** v. 105, n. 3, Jul, p.193- 202. 2003.

CZEH, M.; GRESSENS, P.; KAINDL, A. M. The yin and yang of microglia. **Dev Neurosci,** v. 33,

n. 3-4, p.199-209. 2011.

DEFEO, D. R.; MYERS, P.; FOLTZ, E. L.; EVERETT, B.; RAMSHAW, B. Histological examination of kaolin-induced hydrocephalus. Its implications in the therapy of animals with experimentally induced hydrocephalus. **J Neurosurg,** v. 50, n. 1, Jan, p.70-4.1979.

DEL BIGIO, M. R.; BRUNI, J. E.; FEWER, H. D. Human neonatal hydrocephalus. An electron microscopic study of the periventricular tissue. **J Neurosurg,** v. 63, n. 1, Jul, p.56-63. 1985.

DEL BIGIO, M. R.; KANFER, J. N.; ZHANG, Y. W. Myelination delay in the cerebral white matter of immature rats with kaolin-induced hydrocephalus is reversible. **J Neuropathol Exp Neurol,** v. 56, n. 9, Sep, p.1053-1066. 1997.

DEL BIGIO, M. R.; MCALLISTERII, J. P. Hydrocephalus - Pathology. In: CHOUX, M., DI ROCCO, C. AL, E. Paediatric Neurosurgery. London: Churchill Livingstoneed., 1999, p.217- 236

DEL BIGIO, M. R.; WILSON, M. J.; ENNO, T. Chronic hydrocephalus in rats and humans: white matter loss and behaviour changes. **Ann Neurol,** v. 53, n. 3, Mar, p.337-346. 2003.

DEVARAJ, S.; TANG, R.; ADAMS-HUET, B.; HARRIS, A.; SEENIVASAN, T.; DE LEMOS, J. A.; JIALAL, I. Effect of high-dose alpha-tocopherol supplementation on biomarkers of oxidative stress and inflammation and carotid atherosclerosis in patients with coronary artery disease. **Am J Clin Nutr,** v. 86, n. 5, Nov, p.1392-1398. 2007.

DI CURZIO, D. L.; TURNER-BRANNEN, E.; DEL BIGIO, M. R. Oral antioxidant therapy for juvenile rats with kaolin-induced hydrocephalus. **Fluids Barriers CNS,** v. 11, n., p.23. 2014.

DOHARE, P.; HYZINSKI-GARCIA, M. C.; VIPANI, A.; BOWENS, N. H.; NALWALK, J. W.; FEUSTEL, P. J.; KELLER, R. W., JR.; JOURD'HEUIL, D.; MONGIN, A. A. The neuroprotective properties of the superoxide dismutase mimetic tempol correlate with its ability to reduce pathological glutamate release in a rodent model of stroke. **Free Radiation Biol Med,** v., n., Sep 12. 2014.

DRINGEN, R.; GUTTERER, J. M.; HIRRLINGER, J. Glutathione metabolism in brain metabolic interaction between astrocytes and neurons in the defence against reactive oxygen species. **Eur J Biochem,** v. 267, n. 16, Aug, p.4912-4916. 2000.

EDWARDS, M. S.; HARRISON, M. R.; HALKS-MILLER, M.; NAKAYAMA, D. K.; BERGER, M. S.; GLICK, P. L.; CHINN, D. H. Kaolin-induced congenital hydrocephalus in utero in foetal lambs and rhesus monkeys. **J Neurosurg,** v. 60, n. 1, Jan, p.115-122. 1984.

FERSTEN, E.; GORDON-KRAJCER, W.; GLOWACKI, M.; MROZIAK, B.; JURKIEWICZ, J.; CZERNICKI, Z. Cerebrospinal fluid free-radical peroxidation products and cognitive functioning patterns differentiate varieties of normal pressure hydrocephalus. **Folia Neuropathol,** v. 42, n. 3, p. 133-140. 2004.

GARNE, E.; LOANE, M.; ADDOR, M. C.; BOYD, P. A.; BARISIC, L; DOLK, H. Congenital hydrocephalus-prevalence, prenatal diagnosis and outcome of pregnancy in four European regions. **Eur J Paediatr Neurol,** v. 14, n. 2, Mar, p.150-155. 2010.

GOZZI, M.; NIELSON, D. M.; LENROOT, R. K.; OSTUNI, J. L.; LUCKENBAUGH, D. A.;

THURM, A. E.; GIEDD, J. N.; SWEDO, S. E. A magnetisation transfer imaging study of corpus callosum myelination in young children with autism. **Biol Psychiatry,** v. 72, n. 3, Aug 1, p.215-220. 2012.

HALLIWELL, B.; WHETEMAN, M. Measuring reactive species and oxidative damage in vivo and in cell culture: how should you do it and what do the results mean? **Br J Pharmacol,** v. 142, n. 2004.

HALLIWELL, B. G., J. M. C.. Free Radicals in Biology and Medicine. New York: Oxford. 2007

HIGASHI, Y.; JITSUIKI, D.; CHAYAMA, K.; YOSHIZUMI, M. Edaravone (3-methyl-l- phenyl-2-pyrazolin-5-one), a novel free radical scavenger, for treatment of cardiovascular diseases. **Recent Pat Cardiovasc Drug Discov,** v. 1, n. 1, Jan, p.85-93. 2006.

HOCHWALD, G. M. Animal models of hydrocephalus: recent developments. **Proc Soc Exp Biol Med,** v. 178, n. 1, Jan, p.1-11. 1985.

HU, Q.; VAKHMJANIN, A.; LI, B.; TANG, J.; ZHANG, J. H. Hyperbaric oxygen therapy fails to reduce hydrocephalus formation following subarachnoid haemorrhage in rats. **Med Gas Res,** v. 4, n., p.12. 2014.

INOUE, Y.; YABE, T.; OKADA, K.; NAKAMURA, Y. Effect of Edaravone on acute brainstem-cerebellar infarction with vertigo and sudden hearing loss. **Auris Nasus Larynx,** v. 41, n. 3, Jun, p.303-306. 2014.

ISHIBASHI, A.; YOSHITAKE, Y.; ADACHI, H. Investigation of effect of Edaravone on ischemic stroke. **Kurume Med J,** v. 60, n. 2, p.53-57. 2013.

ISHIKAWA, A.; YOSHIDA, H.; METOKI, N.; TOKI, T.; IMAIZUMI, T.; MATSUMIYA, T.; YAMASHITA, K.; TAIMA, K.; SATOH, K. Edaravone inhibits the expression of vascular endothelial growth factor in human astrocytes exposed to hypoxia. **Neurosci Res,** v. 59, n. 4, Dec, p.406-412. 2007.

ITO, H.; WATE, R.; ZHANG, L; OHNISHI, S.; KANEKO, S.; NAKANO, S.; KUSAKA, H. Treatment with Edaravone, initiated at symptom onset, slows motor decline and decreases SOD1 deposition in ALS mice. **Exp Neurol,** v. 213, n. 2, Oct, p.448-455. 2008.

ITOH, T.; SATOU, T.; NISHIDA, S.; TSUBAKI, M.; HASHIMOTO, S.; ITO, H. The novel free radical scavenger, Edaravone, increases neural stem cell number around the area of damage following rat traumatic brain injury. **Neurotox Res,** v. 16, n. 4, Nov, p.378-389. 2009.

JUCÁ, C. E. B.; LINS NETO, A.; OLIVEIRA, R. S.; MACHADO, H. R. Treatment of hydrocephalus by ventriculoperitoneal shunt: analysis of 150 consecutive cases in the hospital of the faculty of medicine of Ribeirão Preto. **Acta Cir Bras,** v. 17, n., p.59-63. 2002.

JULIAN-REYNIER, C.; PHILIP, N.; SCHEINER, C.; AURRAN, Y.; CHABAL, F.; MARON, A.; GOMBERT, A.; AYME, S. hnpact of prenatal diagnosis by ultrasound on the prevalence of congenital anomalies at birth in southem France. **J Epidemiol Community Health,** v. 48, n. 3, Jun, p.290-296. 1994.

KAMIDA, T.; FUJIKI, M.; OOBA, H.; ANAN, M.; ABE, T.; KOBAYASHI, H. Neuroprotective effects of Edaravone, a free radical scavenger, on the rat hippocampus after pilocarpine-induced status epilepticus. **Seizure,** v. 18, n. 1, Jan, p.71-75. 2009.

KHAN, O. H.; ENNO, T. L.; DEL BIGIO, M. R. Brain damage in neonatal rats following kaolin induction of hydrocephalus. **Exp Neurol,** v. 200, n. 2, Aug, p.311-320. 2006.

KIEFER, M.; EYMANN, R.; VON TILING, S.; MULLER, A.; STEUDEL, W. L; BOOZ, K. H. The ependyma in chronic hydrocephalus. **Childs Nerv Syst,** v. 14, n. 6, Jun, p.263-270. 1998.

KIKUCHI, K.; MIURA, N.; KAWAHARA, K. L; MURAI, Y.; MORIOKA, M.; LAPCHAK, P. A.; TANAKA, E. Edaravone (Radicut), a free radical scavenger, is a potentially useful addition to thrombolytic therapy in patients with acute ischemic stroke. **Biomed Rep,** v. 1, n. 1, Jan, p.7-12. 2013.

LEE, M. J.; MALIAKAL, P.; CHEN, L.; MENG, X.; BONDOC, F. Y.; PRABHU, S.; LAMBERT, G.; MOHR, S.; YANG, C. S. Pharmacokinetics of tea catechins after ingestion of green tea and (-)-epigallocatechin-3-gallate by humans: formation of different metabolites and individual variability. **Cancer Epidemiol Biomarkers Prev,** v. 11, n. 10 Pt 1, Oct, p.1025-1032. 2002.

LI, Q.; BI, M. J.; BI, W. K.; KANG, H.; YAN, L. J.; GUO, Y. L. Edaravone attenuates brain damage in rats after acute CO poisoning through inhibiting apoptosis and oxidative stress. **Environ Toxicol,** v., n., Oct 28. 2014.

LI, X.; LI, L.; LI, J.; SIPPLE, J.; SCHICK, J.; MEHTA, P. A.; DAVIES, S. M.; DASGUPTA, B.; WACLAW, R. R.; PANG, Q. Concomitant Inactivation of Foxo3a and Fancc or Fancd2 Reveals a Two-Tier Protection from Oxidative Stress-Induced Hydrocephalus. **Antioxid Redox Signal**, v., n., Mar 12. 2014.

LOPES, L., S.; SLOBODIAN, L; DEL BIGIO, M. R. Characterisation of juvenile and young adult mice following induction of hydrocephalus with kaolin. **Exp Neurol,** v. 219, n. 1, Sep, p.187-196. 2009.

MABE, H.; SUZUKI, K.; NAGAI, H. Cerebral blood flow after ventriculoperitoneal shunt in children with hydrocephalus. **Childs Nerv Syst,** v. 6, n. 7, Nov, p.388-391. 1990.

MCLONE, D. G. Consensus: modelling of hydrocephalus. **Childs Nerv Syst,** v. 10, n. 1, Jan, p.24-28. 1994.

MILHORAT, T. H. Paediatric Neurosurgery. 2 ed. Philadelphia: F. A. Davis Co. 1979

MORI, K.; MIYAKE, H.; KURISAKA, M.; SAKAMOTO, T. Immunohistochemical localisation of superoxide dismutase in congenital hydrocephalic rat brain. **Childs Nerv Syst,** v. 9, n. 3, Jun, p.136-141. 1993.

MUNAKATA, A.; OHKUMA, H.; NAKANO, T.; SHIMAMURA, N.; ASANO, K.; NARAOKA, M. Effect of a free radical scavenger, Edaravone, in the treatment of patients with aneurysmal subarachnoid haemorrhage. **Neurosurgery,** v. 64, n. 3, Mar, p.423-428; discussion 428-429. 2009.

NAKAMURA, T.; KURODA, Y.; YAMASHITA, S.; ZHANG, X.; MIYAMOTO, O.; TAMIYA, T.; NAGAO, S.; XI, G.; KEEP, R. F.; ITANO, T. Edaravone attenuates brain oedema and neurologic deficits in a rat model of acute intracerebral haemorrhage. **Stroke,** v. 39, n. 2, Feb, p.463-469. 2008.

NEWBOULD, R. D.; NICHOLAS, R.; THOMAS, C. L.; QUEST, R.; LEE, J. S.; HONEYFIELD, L.; COLASANTI, A.; MALIK, O.; MATTOSCIO, M.; MATTHEWS, P. M.; SORMANI, M. P.WALDMAN, A. D.; MURARO, P. A. Age independently affects myelin integrity as detected by magnetisation transfer magnetic resonance imaging in multiple sclerosis. **Neuroimage Clin,** v. 4, n., p.641-648. 2014.

NISHINO, T.; TAMURA, I. The mechanism of conversion of xanthine dehydrogenase to oxidase and the role of the enzyme in reperfusion injury. **Adv Exp Med Biol,** v. 309A, n., p.327-333. 1991.

NOOR, J. L; IKEDA, T.; MISHIMA, K.; AOO, N.; OHTA, S.; EGASHIRA, N.; IWASAKI, K.; FUJIWARA, M.; IKENOUE, T. Short-term administration of a new free radical scavenger, Edaravone, is more effective than its long-term administration for the treatment of neonatal hypoxic-ischemic encephalopathy. **Stroke,** v. 36, n. 11, Nov, p.2468-2474. 2005.

OHTA, Y.; TAKAMATSU, K.; FUKUSHIMA, T.; IKEGAMI, S.; TAKEDA, L; OTA, T.; GOTO, K.; ABE, K. Efficacy of the free radical scavenger, Edaravone, for motor palsy of acute lacunar infarction. **Intern Med,** v. 48, n. 8, p.593-596. 2009.

PEKNY, M.; PEKNA, M. Astrocyte Reactivity and Reactive Astrogliosis: Costs and Benefits. **Physiol Rev,** v. 94, n. 4, Oct, p. 1077-1098. 2014.

PORTNOY, H. D.; BRANCH, C.; CASTRO, M. E. The relationship of intracranial venous pressure to hydrocephalus. **Childs Nerv Syst,** v. 10, n. 1, Jan, p.29-35. 1994.

REN, Y.; WEI, B.; SONG, X.; AN, N.; ZHOU, Y.; JIN, X.; ZHANG, Y. Edaravone's free radical scavenging mechanisms of neuroprotection against cerebral ischemia: review of the literature. **Int J Neurosci,** v., n., Sep 24. 2014.

ROCHA CATALAO, C. H.; LEME CORRÊA, D. A.; BERNARDINO GARCIA, C. A.; DOS SANTOS, A. C.; GARRIDO SALMON, C. E.; ALVES ROCHA, M. J.; DA SILVA LOPES, L. Pre- and postshunting magnetization transfer ratios are in accordance with neurological and behavioural changes in hydrocephalic immature rats. **Dev Neurosci,** v. 36, n. 6, p.520-531. 2014.

SATO, O.; 01, S.; YAMADA, S. Hydrocephalus: experimental considerations and clinical analyses. In: CHOUX, M., DI ROCCO, C., HOCKLEY, A. WALKER, M. Paediatric neurosurgery. London: 1999:237-252.: Churchill Livingstoneed., 1999

SHOESMITH, C. L.; BUIST, R.; DEL BIGIO, M. R. Magnetic resonance imaging study of extracellular fluid tracer movement in brains of immature rats with hydrocephalus. **Neurol Res,** v. 22, n. 1, Jan, p.111-116. 2000.

SHOKRZADEH, M.; SHAKI, F.; MOHAMMADI, E.; REZAGHOLIZADEH, N.; EBRAHIMI, F. Edaravone decreases paraquat toxicity in a549 cells and lung isolated mitochondria. **Iran J Pharm Res,** v. 13, n. 2, Spring, p.675-681. 2014.

SIES, H. Oxidative stress: oxidants and antioxidants. **Exp Physiol,** v. 82, n. 2, Mar, p.291- 295. 1997.

SIESJO, B. K.; AGARDH, C. D.; BENGTSSON, F. Free radicals and brain damage. **Cerebrovasc**

Brain Metab Rev, v. 1, n. 3, Fali, p.165-211. 1989.

TATEM, K. S.; QUINN, J. L.; PHADKE, A.; YU, Q.; GORDISH-DRESSMAN, H.; NAGARAJU, K. Behavioural and locomotor measurements using an open field activity monitoring system for skeletal muscle diseases. **J Vis Exp,** v., n. 91. 2014.

TOYODA, K.; FUJII, K.; KAMOUCHI, M.; NAKANE, H.; ARIHIRO, S.; OKADA, Y.; IBAYASHI, S.; HDA, M. Free radical scavenger, Edaravone, in stroke with internal carotid artery occlusion. **J Neurol Sei,** v. 221, n. 1-2, Jun 15, p.11-17. 2004.

TSURUOKA, A.; ATSUMI, C.; MIZUKAMI, H.; IMAI, T.; HAGIWARA, Y.; HASEGAWA, Y. Effects of Edaravone, a Free Radical Scavenger, on Circulating Levels of MMP-9 and Hemorrhagic Transformation in Patients with Intravenous Thrombolysis Using Low-dose Alteplase. **J Stroke Cerebrovasc Dis,** v., n., Oct 1. 2014.

VOGEL, P.; READ, R. W.; HANSEN, G. M.; PAYNE, B. J.; SMALL, D.; SANDS, A. T.; ZAMBROWICZ, B. P. Congenital hydrocephalus in genetically engineered mice. **Vet Pathol,** v. 49, n. 1, Jan, p.166-181. 2012.

WANG, G. H.; JIANG, Z. L.; LI, Y. C.; LI, X.; SHI, H.; GAO, Y. Q.; VOSLER, P. S.; CHEN, J. Free-radical scavenger Edaravone treatment confers neuroprotection against traumatic brain injury in rats. **J Neurotrauma,** v. 28, n. 10, Oct, p.2123-2134. 2011.

WANG, J.; GUO, G.; WANG, W.; TANG, Y.; SHUN, J.; ZHOU, X.; ZHANG, P. Effect of methylprednisolone and Edaravone administration on spinal cord injury. **Eur Rev Med Pharmacol Sei,** v. 17, n. 20, Oct, p.2766-2772. 2013.

WATANABE, T.; TAHARA, M.; TODO, S. The novel antioxidant Edaravone: from bench to bedside. **Cardiovasc Ther,** v. 26, n. 2, Summer, p.101-114. 2008.

WU, T. W.; ZENG, L. H.; WU, J.; FUNG, K. P. MCI-186: further histochemical and biochemical evidence of neuroprotection. **Life Sei,** v. 67, n. 19, Sep 29, p.2387-2392. 2000.

YAGI, K.; KITAZATO, K. T.; UNO, M.; TADA, Y.; KINOUCHI, T.; SHIMADA, K.; NAGAHIRO, S. Edaravone, a free radical scavenger, inhibits MMP-9-related brain haemorrhage in rats treated with tissue plasminogen activator. **Stroke,** v. 40, n. 2, Feb, p.626- 631. 2009.

YAMADA, H.; YOKOTA, A.; FURUTA, A.; HORIE, A. Reconstitution of shunted mantle in experimental hydrocephalus. **J Neurosurg,** v. 76, n. 5, May, p.856-862. 1992.

YOSHIDA, H.; YANAI, H.; NAMIKI, Y.; FUKATSU-SASAKI, K.; FURUTANI, N.; TADA, N. Neuroprotective effects of Edaravone: a novel free radical scavenger in cerebrovascular injury. **CNS Drug Rev,** v. 12, n. 1, Spring, p.9-20. 2006.

YUAN, W.; MANGANO, F. T.; AIR, E. L.; HOLLAND, S. K.; JONES, B. V.; ALTAYE, M.; BIERBRAUER, K. Anisotropic diffusion properties in infants with hydrocephalus: a diffusion tensor imaging study. **AJNR Am J Neuroradiol,** v. 30, n. 9, Oct, p. 1792-1798. 2009.

ZAARAOUI, W.; DELOIRE, M.; MERLE, M.; GIRARD, C.; RAFFARD, G.; BIRAN, M.; INGLESE, M.; PETRY, K. G.; GONEN, O.; BROCHET, B.; FRANCONI, J. M.; DOUSSET, V.

Monitoring demyelination and remyelination by magnetisation transfer imaging in the mouse brain at 9.4 T. **MAGMA,** v. 21, n. 5, Sep, p.357-362. 2008.

ZAGER, E. L.; AMES, A., 3RD. Reduction of cellular energy requirements. Screening for agents that may protect against CNS ischemia. **J Neurosurg,** v. 69, n. 4, Oct, p.568-579. 1988.

ZHANG, N.; KOMINE-KOBAYASHI, M.; TANAKA, R.; LIU, M.; MIZUNO, Y.; URABE, T. Edaravone reduces early accumulation of oxidative products and sequential inflammatory responses after transient focal ischemia in mice brain. **Stroke,** v. 36, n. 10, Oct, p.2220-2225. 2005.

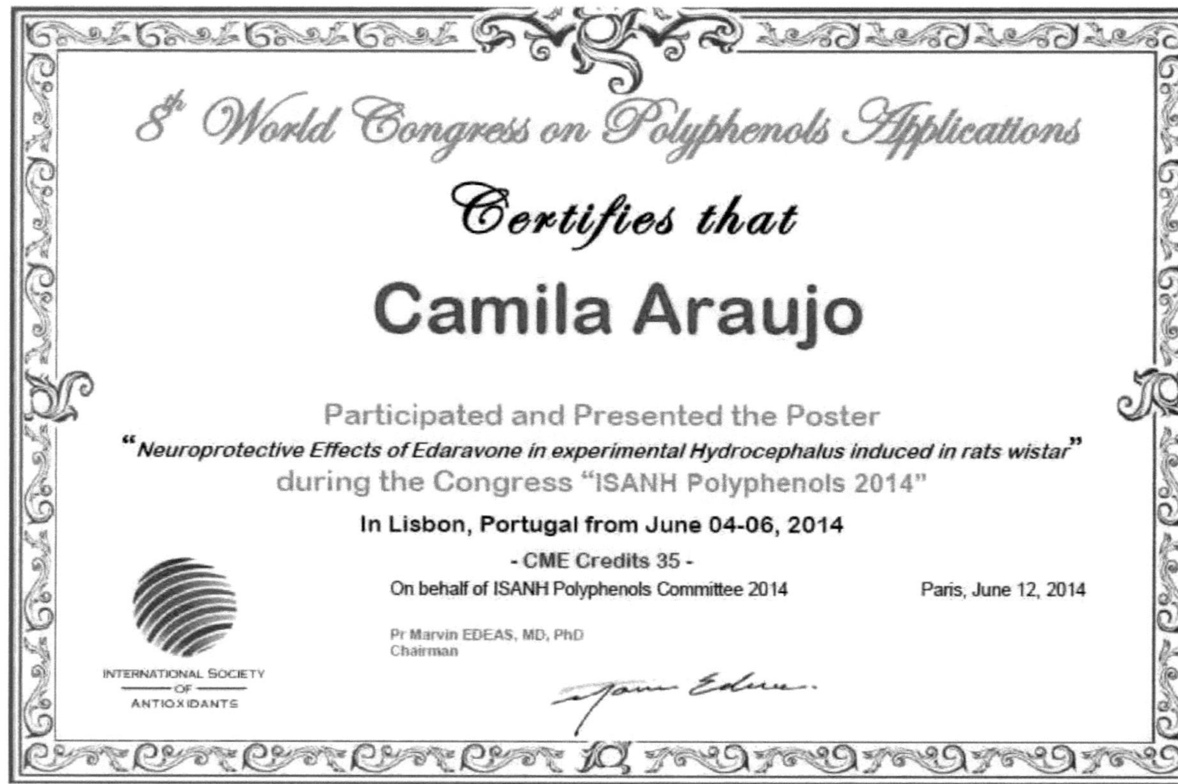

ANEXOS

8th World Congress on Polyphenols Applications

Certifies that

Camila Araujo

Participated and Presented the Poster

“Neuroprotective Effects of Edaravone in experimental Hydrocephalus induced in rats wistar”

during the Congress “ISANH Polyphenols 2014”

In Lisbon, Portugal from June 04-06, 2014

- CME Credits 35 -

On behalf of ISANH Polyphenols Committee 2014

Paris, June 12, 2014

Pr Marvin EDEAS, MD, PhD
Chairman

INTERNATIONAL SOCIETY OF ANTIOXIDANTS

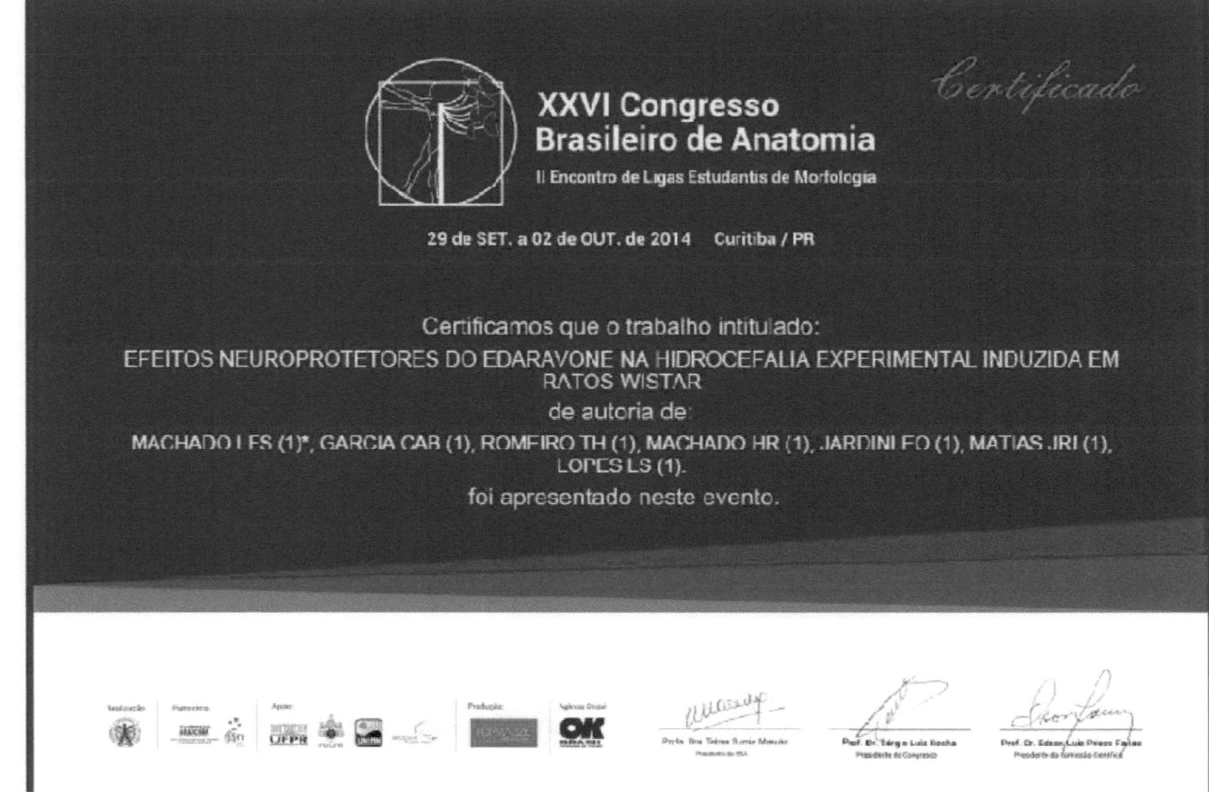
Certificado
XXVI Congresso
Brasileiro de Anatomia
II Encontro de Ligas Estudantis de Morfologia
29 de SET. a 02 de OUT. de 2014 Curitiba / PR
Certificamos que o trabalho intitulado:
EFEITOS NEUROPROTETORES DO EDARAVONE NA HIDROCEFALIA EXPERIMENTAL INDUZIDA EM RATOS WISTAR
de autoria de:
MACHADO LFS (1)*, GARCIA CAB (1), ROMEIRO TH (1), MACHADO HR (1), JARDINI EO (1), MATIAS JRI (1), LOPES LS (1).
foi apresentado neste evento.

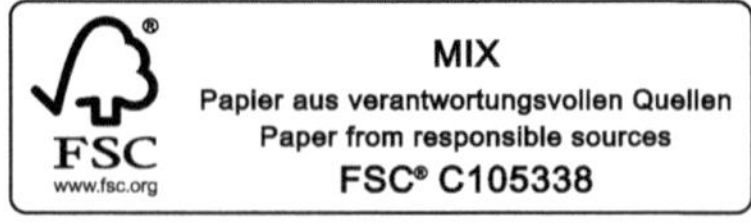

Printed by Books on Demand GmbH, Norderstedt / Germany